HERBAL GUIDE

BOOK

FOR BEGINNERS

Explore the Healing Power in Natural Medicinal Plants for Common Ailments to Improve your Wellness Including Health Benefits and More

DR. GARY C. WONG

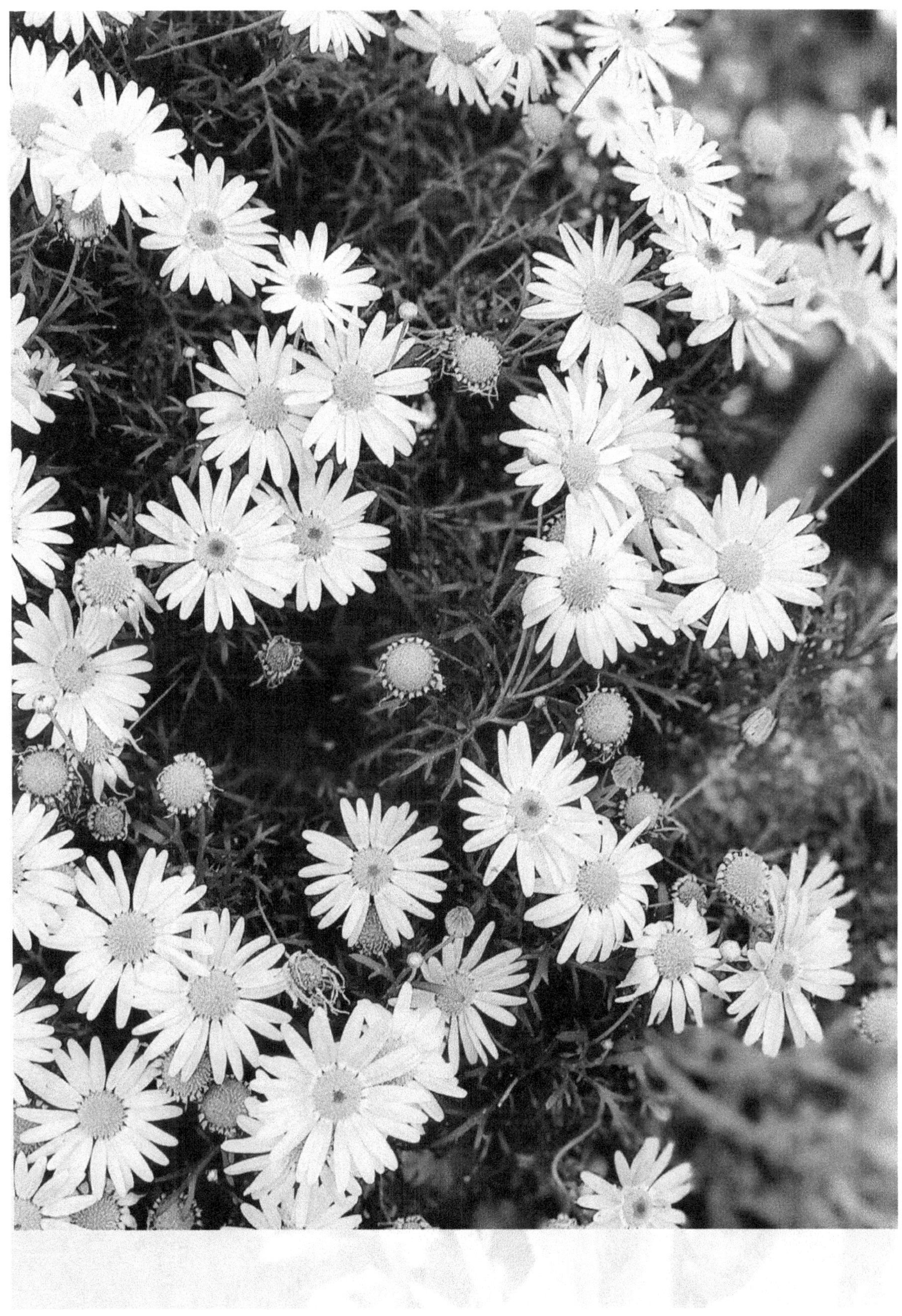

Copyright: © 2024 by Dr. Gary C. Wong

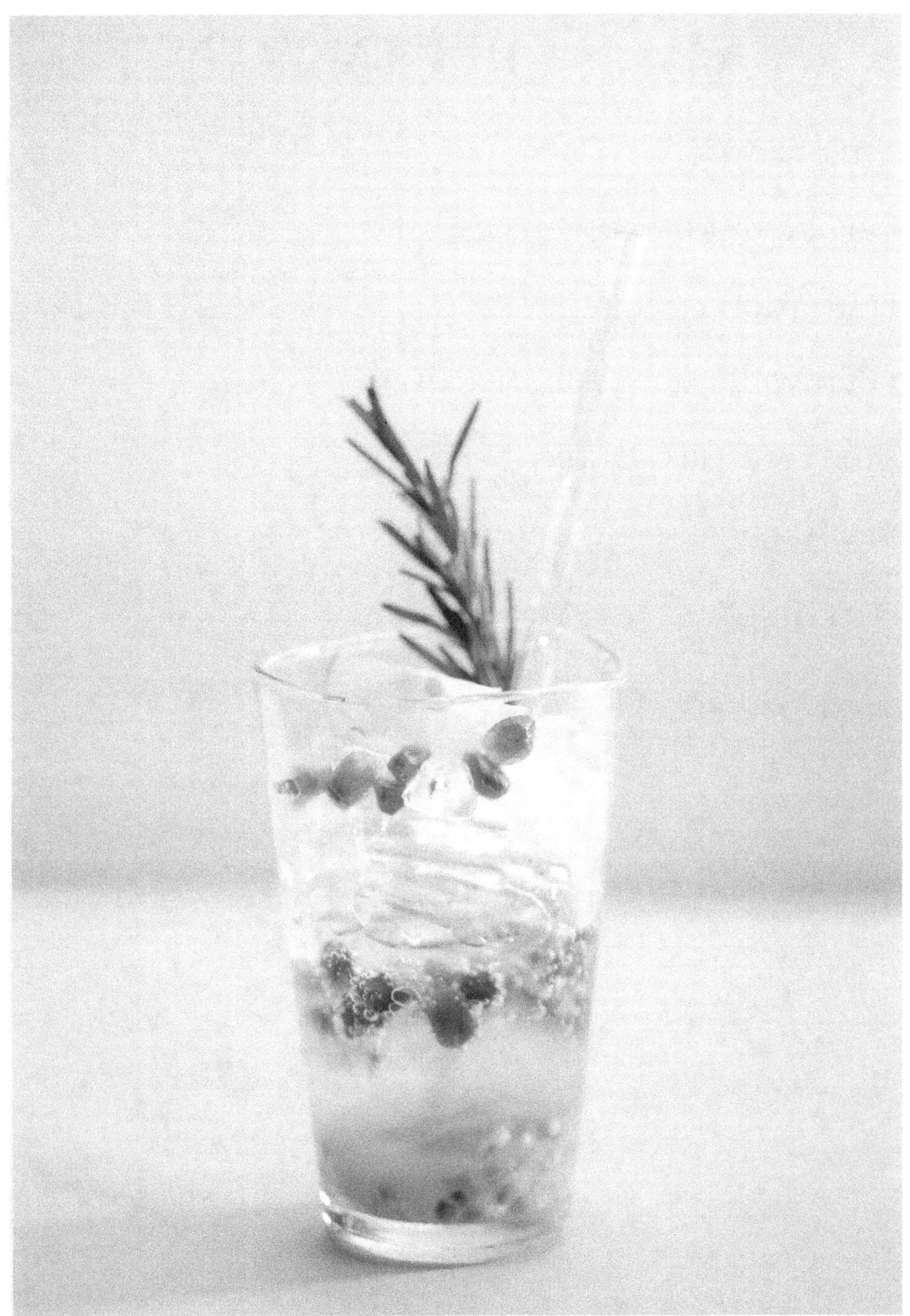

TABLE OF CONTENT

INTRODUCTION

Herbalism, the practice of using plants for their medicinal properties, has been an integral part of human history for millennia. Long before the advent of modern pharmaceuticals, our ancestors turned to the natural world for healing and sustenance. The wisdom they gathered over centuries has been passed down through generations, evolving with the times yet retaining its core essence: a profound respect for the healing power of nature.

History and Philosophy of Herbalism

The roots of herbalism reach deep into the past, intertwining with the earliest human civilizations. Ancient texts from China, Egypt, Greece, and India reveal sophisticated herbal practices that laid the groundwork for modern medicine. The Ebers Papyrus, a medical document from ancient Egypt dated around 1550 BCE, lists over 850 herbal medicines. In ancient China, the Shen Nong Ben Cao Jing, written around 2800 BCE, details the use of 365 medicinal plants.

Greek physician Hippocrates, often called the "father of medicine," emphasized the healing power of nature. His holistic approach to health, which combined diet, exercise, and herbal remedies, resonates with modern herbalism's philosophy. Similarly, the Roman physician Galen developed extensive herbal preparations that influenced medical practices for centuries.

In the East, traditional systems like Ayurveda and Traditional Chinese Medicine (TCM) have harnessed the power of herbs for thousands of years. Ayurveda, originating in India over 3,000 years ago, classifies herbs according to their effects on the body's doshas (vital energies). TCM employs a sophisticated system of diagnosis and treatment, using herbs to balance the body's qi (vital energy).

The Middle Ages in Europe saw the rise of monastic gardens, where monks cultivated medicinal plants and preserved herbal knowledge through texts like the "Physica" by Hildegard of Bingen. During the Renaissance, herbalism experienced a revival as scholars rediscovered ancient texts and botanists explored the medicinal properties of plants.

Despite the rise of synthetic drugs in the 20th century, herbalism has persisted, driven by a growing interest in natural and holistic health approaches. Today, herbalism is experiencing a resurgence, fueled by an increasing awareness of the limitations and side effects of modern pharmaceuticals and a desire to reconnect with nature.

The Benefits and Risks of Herbal Remedies

Herbal remedies offer numerous benefits, making them a valuable addition to modern healthcare. They are generally more affordable than synthetic drugs and often come with fewer side effects. Many herbs provide a broad spectrum of benefits, supporting overall health and well-being in addition to addressing specific ailments. For instance, turmeric is not only anti-inflammatory but also antioxidant and supports liver health.

Herbs often work gently and synergistically with the body's natural processes. They can support and strengthen the body's own healing mechanisms, providing a holistic approach to health. This makes herbal remedies particularly suitable for chronic conditions and for preventive health care.

Moreover, the use of herbal remedies can promote a closer connection with nature. Growing and preparing herbs encourages a deeper understanding and appreciation of the natural world, fostering a sense of self-reliance and empowerment in managing one's health.

However, it is crucial to recognize that herbal remedies are not without risks. Misidentification of plants, incorrect dosages, and potential interactions with pharmaceutical drugs can lead to adverse effects. For example, while St. John's Wort is effective for mild to moderate depression, it can interact dangerously with various medications, including antidepressants, birth control pills, and blood thinners.

Additionally, the quality and potency of herbal products can vary widely. Factors such as growing conditions, harvesting practices, and processing methods can all influence an herb's effectiveness. It is essential to use high-quality, reputable sources for herbal products and to consult with a knowledgeable healthcare provider, especially when dealing with serious health conditions or when combining herbal remedies with conventional treatments.

Understanding Herbal Medicine: Traditional vs. Modern Approaches

Herbal medicine stands at the crossroads of traditional wisdom and modern science. Traditional herbalism, rooted in centuries of empirical observation and cultural practices, offers a holistic perspective on health. It considers the individual as a whole, taking into account physical, emotional, and spiritual aspects. Traditional systems like Ayurveda, TCM, and Native American medicine emphasize the balance and harmony of the body's energies and the interconnectedness of all life.

Modern herbalism, while deeply influenced by these traditional practices, also incorporates scientific research and evidence-based methods. Advances in pharmacology and chemistry have enabled a deeper understanding of the active compounds in plants and their mechanisms of action. This scientific validation has helped to integrate herbal medicine into mainstream healthcare, enhancing its credibility and acceptance.

One of the key differences between traditional and modern approaches lies in the use of whole plants versus isolated compounds. Traditional herbalism typically employs whole plants or complex mixtures, which are believed to work synergistically to enhance therapeutic effects and minimize side effects. For instance, the whole echinacea plant is used to boost the immune system, rather than isolating a single active ingredient.

Modern medicine, on the other hand, often focuses on isolating and synthesizing specific compounds. This approach has led to the development of powerful pharmaceuticals derived from plants, such as aspirin from willow bark and digitalis from foxglove. While this method can produce potent and targeted treatments, it may also increase the risk of side effects and diminish the holistic benefits of the whole plant.

Despite these differences, there is a growing convergence between traditional and modern herbalism. Integrative medicine, which combines conventional and complementary therapies, is gaining traction. This approach seeks to harness the best of both worlds, using evidence-based herbal remedies alongside conventional treatments to support health and healing.

The future of herbal medicine lies in this integrative approach. Continued research and clinical trials are essential to validate traditional practices, ensure safety, and discover new therapeutic applications. By bridging the gap between ancient wisdom and modern science, we can create a more comprehensive and holistic healthcare system.

1

Getting Started with Herbalism

Embarking on the journey of herbalism opens the door to a world where nature's bounty becomes your ally in health and wellness. This chapter, "Getting Started with Herbalism," is designed to be your first step into understanding the basic principles and practices of this ancient, yet ever-relevant field.

Herbalism, at its core, involves the use of plants and their extracts for medicinal purposes. This practice, steeped in centuries of tradition, marries the wisdom of ancient healers with modern scientific insights, offering a holistic approach to health. Whether you are driven by a desire to take control of your wellness naturally or to deepen your connection with the environment, this chapter will equip you with the foundational knowledge needed to begin your herbalist journey.

We will start by familiarizing you with basic herbal terminology, ensuring that you can confidently navigate the language of herbalism. Understanding these terms will demystify the process and enhance your ability to learn and communicate about herbs effectively.

Next, we will delve into the essential tools and equipment every budding herbalist should have. From the must-have items in your herbal toolkit to tips on selecting the right equipment, this section will prepare you to work with herbs efficiently and safely.

Finally, we will explore the critical aspect of sourcing quality herbs. You'll learn about wildcrafting—harvesting plants from their natural habitats—and the considerations involved in ensuring this practice is sustainable and ethical. Additionally, we'll cover how to purchase high-quality herbs, ensuring you always have the best ingredients for your remedies.

By the end of this chapter, you will have a solid foundation to build upon, ready to delve deeper into the fascinating and rewarding practice of herbalism. Whether you're growing your own herbs or sourcing them from trusted suppliers, this initial step will set you on the path to becoming a knowledgeable and confident herbalist.

Basic Herbal Terminology

Understanding the language of herbalism is crucial for any beginner. This section introduces you to the key terms and concepts that form the backbone of herbal practice.

1. **Adaptogens:** These are herbs that help the body adapt to stress and restore balance. Examples include ashwagandha, rhodiola, and holy basil.
2. **Analgesic:** An herb that relieves pain. Willow bark and turmeric are common examples.
3. **Antioxidants:** Compounds found in herbs that protect the body from damage caused by free radicals. Green tea and rosemary are rich in antioxidants.
4. **Astringent:** Herbs that cause the contraction of tissues, often used to reduce bleeding or treat skin conditions. Witch hazel and yarrow are notable astringents.
5. **Carminative:** Herbs that relieve gas and bloating by soothing the digestive tract. Peppermint and fennel fall into this category.
6. **Decoction:** A method of extraction by boiling tough plant materials like roots or bark to obtain their medicinal properties.
7. **Infusion:** Similar to making tea, this method involves steeping delicate plant parts like leaves or flowers in hot water to extract their beneficial compounds.
8. **Poultice:** A soft, moist mass of plant material applied directly to the skin to treat wounds or inflammation.
9. **Tincture:** A concentrated herbal extract made by soaking herbs in alcohol or vinegar.

Familiarizing yourself with these terms will help you navigate herbal literature and communicate more effectively with other herbalists.

Essential Tools and Equipment for Herbalists

Just as a chef needs the right kitchen tools, an herbalist requires specific equipment to prepare and utilize herbs effectively. Here is a list of essential tools and their uses:

1. **Mortar and Pestle:** Used for grinding and crushing herbs to release their active compounds.
2. **Scales:** Precise measurement of herbs is critical for creating effective and safe remedies. Digital scales that measure in grams are ideal.
3. **Jars and Containers:** Glass jars with airtight seals are perfect for storing dried herbs, tinctures, and infusions, protecting them from moisture and light.
4. **Herb Drying Rack:** For those who harvest their own

herbs, a drying rack is essential to air-dry herbs properly.

5. **Labels and Markers:** Keeping track of your herbal preparations is crucial. Always label your jars with the name of the herb, date of preparation, and any other relevant information.

6. **Cheesecloth or Strainer:** Used for straining plant material from infusions, decoctions, and tinctures.

7. **Saucepan and Double Boiler:** Necessary for making infusions, decoctions, and herbal oils.

8. **Dropper Bottles:** For storing and dispensing tinctures and other liquid extracts.

Having the right tools at your disposal will make the process of preparing and using herbs more efficient and enjoyable.

Sourcing Quality Herbs: Wildcrafting vs. Purchasing

The quality of the herbs you use in your preparations is paramount. There are two primary methods for sourcing herbs: wildcrafting and purchasing. Each has its advantages and considerations.

Wildcrafting:

Wildcrafting involves harvesting plants from their natural habitat. This method can be highly rewarding as it connects you directly with nature and ensures that you have control over the quality of the herbs you gather. Here are some guidelines for ethical wildcrafting:

- ➢ **Identification:** Properly identify plants to avoid harvesting the wrong species, which can be ineffective or even harmful.

- ➢ **Sustainability:** Harvest in a way that does not harm the plant population or ecosystem. Take only what you need and leave enough for the plant to continue thriving.

- ➢ **Location:** Avoid areas that may be contaminated with pesticides, pollutants, or heavy metals. National parks, nature reserves, and private lands often have regulations, so ensure you have permission to harvest.

- ➢ **Timing:** Harvest herbs at the optimal time for potency. For example, flowers are best collected when they are in full bloom, while roots are typically harvested in the fall.

Purchasing:

For those who may not have access to wild areas or prefer the convenience, purchasing herbs is a viable alternative. Here are tips for sourcing high-quality herbs:

- ➢ **Reputable Suppliers:** Purchase from established companies known for their quality control and ethical sourcing practices.
- ➢ **Organic Certification:** Look for organic herbs to ensure they are free from pesticides and chemical residues.
- ➢ **Freshness:** Check the packaging date and choose suppliers who offer fresh stock. Herbs lose potency over time, so fresher is better.
- ➢ **Transparency:** Reliable suppliers provide information about the herb's origin, harvesting methods, and processing practices.

Whether you choose to wildcraft or purchase your herbs, ensuring their quality is crucial for making effective and safe herbal remedies.

2

Plant Profiles

Plants are remarkable living organisms that play a vital role in the health and well-being of our planet and its inhabitants. As you delve into the world of herbalism, understanding the unique characteristics and uses of various medicinal plants becomes essential. This section, dedicated to plant profiles, serves as your gateway to appreciating and utilizing the healing properties of herbs.

The chapter begins with an essential skill for any herbalist: the ability to accurately identify medicinal plants. Recognizing different species and understanding their specific traits ensures safe and effective use. Through detailed descriptions and visual guides, you will learn to distinguish between beneficial herbs and potential look-alikes, enhancing your confidence in wildcrafting and gardening.

Next, we explore the various parts of plants used in herbal remedies. From leaves and flowers to roots and seeds, each component offers distinct medicinal properties. By understanding which parts are used and how they contribute to overall health, you can make more informed decisions when preparing herbal treatments.

Each plant profile in this chapter provides comprehensive information on identification, parts used, cultivation, properties, and uses. You will discover the rich history and traditional uses of well-known herbs like chamomile, lavender, and peppermint, as well as lesser-known but equally valuable plants. Detailed cultivation tips will guide you in growing your herbal garden, whether in a small urban space or a sprawling outdoor plot.

Properties and uses are the heart of each plant profile. Here, you will find insights into the therapeutic benefits of each herb, backed by both traditional knowledge and modern research. Whether seeking remedies for common ailments or looking to enhance your culinary creations, the information provided will help you harness the full potential of these natural treasures.

As you progress through the plant profiles, you will build a solid foundation of herbal knowledge. This chapter aims to inspire and educate, fostering a deeper connection to the plants that have supported human health for centuries. With each profile, you gain not just information, but also a greater appreciation for the wisdom and power of nature's pharmacy.

How to Identify Medicinal Plants

Learning to identify medicinal plants is a foundational skill for any herbalist. Whether you are exploring the wilderness or cultivating a garden, accurate plant identification ensures safety and effectiveness in herbal practice. Here are key steps to help you identify medicinal plants with confidence:

- ➢ **Field Guides and Resources:** Invest in reliable field guides specific to your region or seek guidance from reputable online resources. These references provide detailed descriptions, photographs, and illustrations to aid in plant identification.
- ➢ **Botanical Characteristics:** Pay attention to botanical features such as leaves, flowers, stems, and fruits. Understanding the unique characteristics of each plant family and species is crucial. For example, the mint family (Lamiaceae) is known for its square stems and aromatic leaves.
- ➢ **Habitat and Growing Conditions:** Consider where the plant thrives. Some medicinal plants prefer moist, shady environments (e.g., goldenseal), while others thrive in sunny, dry conditions (e.g., echinacea). Understanding habitat preferences enhances your ability to locate specific plants.
- ➢ **Seasonal Cycles:** Plants exhibit distinct growth patterns throughout the year. Learn to recognize plants during different seasons, noting changes in foliage, flowering times, and fruiting periods.
- ➢ **Safety Precautions:** Exercise caution when identifying plants, especially those with toxic look-alikes. Confirm identification using multiple sources and consult with experienced herbalists or botanists if uncertain.

By honing your observational skills and utilizing reliable resources, you will develop proficiency in identifying medicinal plants, unlocking the vast potential of nature's pharmacy.

Guide to Parts of the Plant Used in Remedies

Understanding which parts of medicinal plants to harvest and utilize is essential for creating effective herbal remedies. Different plant parts contain varying concentrations of active compounds and are used accordingly. Here's a guide to commonly used plant parts in herbalism:

➢ **Leaves:** Often rich in volatile oils, vitamins, and minerals, leaves are versatile and commonly used in teas, infusions, and topical preparations. Examples include peppermint leaves for digestive teas and comfrey leaves for skin salves.

➢ **Flowers:** Flowers are prized for their beauty and therapeutic properties. They are often used to make aromatic and soothing herbal teas, as well as infused oils and tinctures. Chamomile flowers, for instance, are renowned for their calming effects.

➢ **Stems and Bark:** Stems and bark may contain potent medicinal compounds, such as alkaloids and tannins. They are utilized in decoctions, which involve simmering the plant material to extract these compounds. Willow bark, containing salicin, is a classic example used for pain relief.

➢ **Roots:** Roots are prized for their concentrated medicinal properties. They are typically harvested in the fall or early spring when the plant's energy is concentrated in the roots. Ginseng root, known for its adaptogenic properties, is a valuable example used in herbal tonics and tinctures.

➢ **Seeds and Fruits:** Seeds and fruits often contain essential oils, antioxidants, and fatty acids. They are used in culinary herbalism and to create medicinal oils and extracts. Examples include flax seeds for their omega-3 fatty acids and elderberries for immune-boosting syrups.

Each plant part offers unique benefits and requires specific harvesting and preparation methods to maximize efficacy. By understanding these nuances, you can harness the full potential of medicinal plants in your herbal practice.

Plant Profile: Aloe Vera

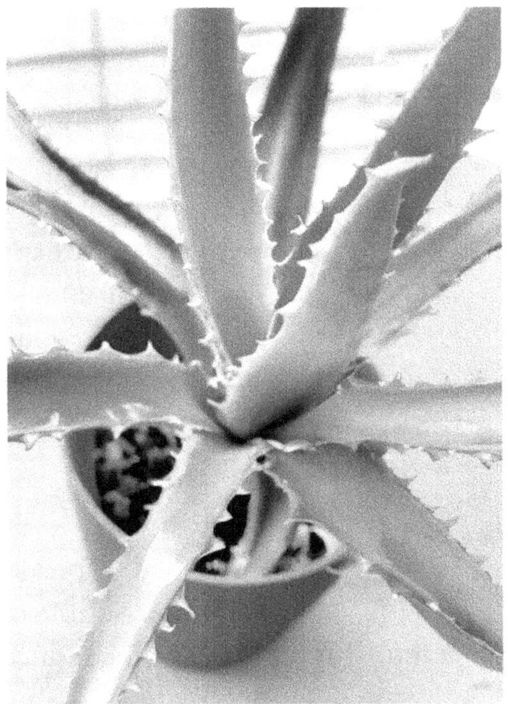

Aloe vera, revered for centuries for its versatile medicinal properties, is a succulent plant that belongs to the genus Aloe. This plant, characterized by its thick, fleshy leaves lined with serrated edges, thrives in arid climates and is renowned for its therapeutic benefits. In this profile, we explore the identification, parts used, cultivation, properties, and uses of aloe vera.

Identification

> **Appearance:** Aloe vera features rosettes of thick, lance-shaped leaves that grow from the base. The leaves are typically green to gray-green, with white spots on the upper and lower surfaces. They can reach lengths of up to 18-24 inches and are edged with small, sharp teeth.

> **Flowers:** Mature aloe vera plants produce tall stalks bearing tubular yellow or orange flowers during the summer months. These flowers attract pollinators and add ornamental value to the plant.

Parts Used

> **Gel:** The inner gel, found within the leaf's thick, succulent tissue, is the most valued part of the plant for its medicinal properties. It is clear and viscous, containing water, vitamins, enzymes, amino acids, and minerals such as calcium, magnesium, and potassium.

> **Latex:** Known as aloe latex or aloe juice, this yellowish-brown substance is found just beneath the plant's skin. It contains anthraquinones, which have strong laxative effects and are used in specific medicinal preparations.

Cultivation

Aloe vera is relatively easy to cultivate, making it a popular choice for home gardens and commercial cultivation in warm, dry climates. Here are key cultivation tips:

- ➢ **Light:** Aloe vera thrives in bright, indirect sunlight. Place it near a sunny window indoors or in a sunny spot outdoors, avoiding direct sunlight, which can cause leaf burn.
- ➢ **Soil:** Use well-draining soil with a sandy or rocky texture to prevent waterlogging, as aloe vera roots are susceptible to rot in overly moist conditions.
- ➢ **Watering:** Allow the soil to dry out completely between waterings. Water deeply but infrequently, especially in winter when the plant is dormant.
- ➢ **Temperature:** Aloe vera prefers temperatures between 55-80°F (13-27°C). Protect it from frost and extreme cold, as prolonged exposure can damage the leaves.

Properties

- ➢ **Anti-inflammatory:** Aloe vera gel contains compounds like acemannan that exhibit anti-inflammatory effects, making it beneficial for soothing irritated skin and reducing inflammation internally when consumed.
- ➢ **Antioxidant:** The gel is rich in antioxidants such as vitamins A, C, and E, which help neutralize free radicals and protect cells from oxidative damage.
- ➢ **Wound Healing:** Aloe vera accelerates wound healing due to its antimicrobial properties and ability to stimulate cell regeneration. It is commonly used to treat burns, cuts, and minor skin abrasions.
- ➢ **Digestive Aid:** Aloe latex acts as a potent laxative, promoting bowel movements and alleviating constipation when used appropriately.

Uses

- ➢ **Skin Care:** Applied topically, aloe vera gel soothes sunburns, moisturizes dry skin, reduces acne inflammation, and promotes overall skin health.
- ➢ **Hair Care:** Aloe vera gel nourishes the scalp, reduces dandruff, and conditions hair, leaving it smooth and shiny.
- ➢ **Internal Health:** When consumed as a juice or supplement (carefully, due to its laxative effects), aloe vera promotes digestive health, boosts immunity, and supports overall well-being.
- ➢ **Cosmetic Applications:** Aloe vera is a common ingredient in cosmetics and skincare products, including lotions, creams, and face masks, due to its moisturizing and soothing properties.

Aloe vera's remarkable versatility and effectiveness in promoting health and well-being have earned it a cherished place in both traditional herbal medicine and modern skincare and wellness practices. Whether grown at home or sourced commercially, this plant continues to be celebrated for its myriad benefits, enhancing both external beauty and internal vitality.

Plant Profile: Chamomile

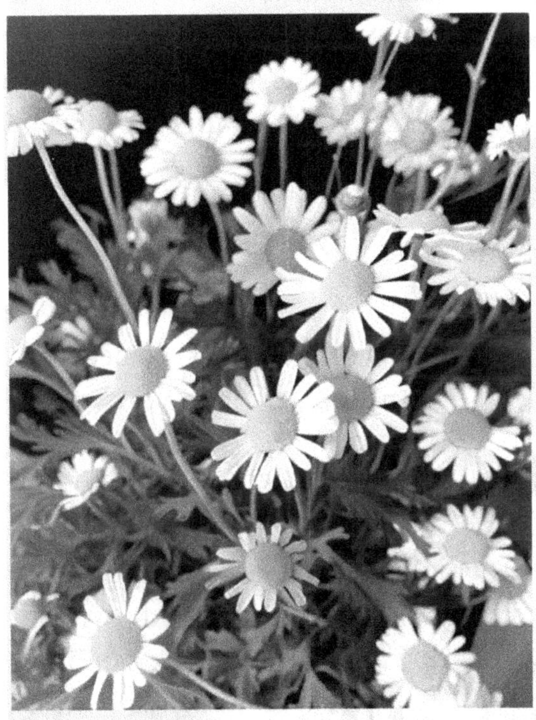

Chamomile, a beloved herb revered for its calming properties and gentle efficacy, belongs to the Asteraceae family and encompasses several species, including German chamomile (Matricaria chamomilla) and Roman chamomile (Chamaemelum nobile). In this profile, we delve into the identification, parts used, cultivation, properties, and diverse uses of chamomile, highlighting its role as a cornerstone of herbal medicine.

Identification

> **Appearance:** Chamomile is characterized by feathery, finely divided leaves that are fern-like in appearance. The plant typically grows low to the ground, forming dense, bushy clumps. The flowers, which bloom in summer, are daisy-like with white petals and a yellow center.
> **Scent:** Chamomile flowers emit a distinct, sweet, apple-like fragrance when crushed, adding to their allure and charm.

Parts Used

> **Flowers:** The flowers of chamomile are the primary part used for medicinal purposes. They are harvested when fully open and dried quickly to preserve their essential oils and therapeutic properties. The flowers contain volatile oils, flavonoids (such as apigenin), and other beneficial compounds.

Cultivation

Chamomile is relatively easy to cultivate, thriving in sunny locations with well-draining soil. Here are key cultivation tips:

- **Light:** Chamomile prefers full sun but can tolerate partial shade, especially in hotter climates.
- **Soil:** Use well-draining, sandy loam soil with a slightly acidic to neutral pH (around 5.6 to 7.5).
- **Watering:** Water regularly to keep the soil moist, especially during dry spells. Avoid overwatering, as chamomile is susceptible to root rot in waterlogged conditions.
- **Propagation:** Chamomile can be propagated from seeds or by dividing existing plants. Directly sow seeds in the garden after the last frost date or start seeds indoors and transplant seedlings once established.

Properties

- **Anti-inflammatory:** Chamomile possesses anti-inflammatory properties that help reduce inflammation and promote healing, making it beneficial for skin conditions, digestive issues, and respiratory ailments.
- **Sedative:** The herb is renowned for its mild sedative effects, promoting relaxation and aiding in sleep when consumed as a tea or used in aromatherapy.
- **Antispasmodic:** Chamomile relaxes smooth muscle tissue, making it effective in easing muscle spasms, menstrual cramps, and gastrointestinal discomfort.
- **Antioxidant:** Rich in antioxidants such as flavonoids, chamomile helps protect cells from oxidative stress and supports overall health.

Uses

- **Digestive Health:** Chamomile tea is a popular remedy for soothing digestive upset, including indigestion, bloating, and gas. It promotes digestion and relieves gastrointestinal spasms.
- **Skin Care:** Applied topically or used in baths, chamomile helps soothe skin irritations, eczema, and minor wounds. It can also lighten dark circles under the eyes.
- **Sleep Aid:** Chamomile tea is consumed before bedtime to promote relaxation and improve sleep quality. It is gentle enough for children and adults alike.
- **Hair Care:** Chamomile infusion or extract is used to enhance hair shine and lighten hair color naturally, especially for blonde hair.

Chamomile's versatility and gentle nature make it a cherished ally in both traditional herbal medicine and modern wellness practices. Whether enjoyed as a calming tea, applied topically for skin care, or used for its digestive benefits, chamomile continues to captivate with its soothing aroma and profound healing properties.

Plant Profile: Echinacea

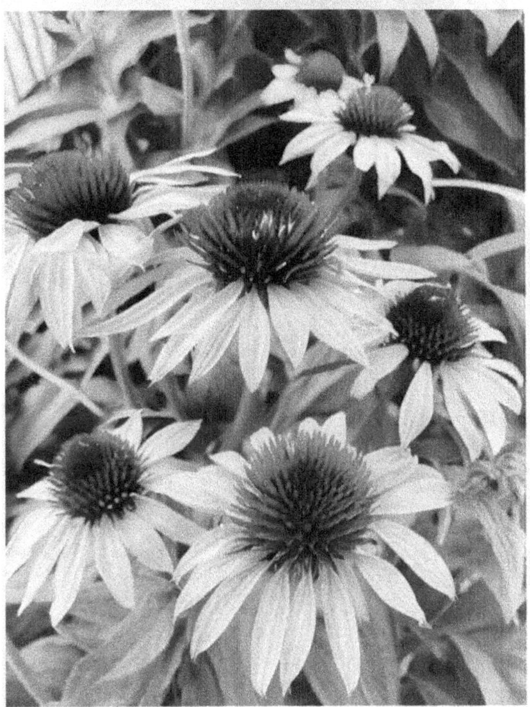

Echinacea, celebrated for its immune-boosting properties and vibrant flowers, belongs to the Asteraceae family and comprises several species, including Echinacea purpurea and Echinacea angustifolia. In this profile, we explore the identification, parts used, cultivation, properties, and diverse uses of echinacea, highlighting its role as a cornerstone of herbal medicine.

Identification

> **Appearance:** Echinacea plants are characterized by sturdy stems that bear large, daisy-like flowers with prominent raised centers (cones). The flowers can range in color from pink and purple to white, depending on the species and variety.

> **Leaves:** Echinacea leaves are lance-shaped, rough-textured, and arranged alternately along the stem. They can be hairy and have serrated edges.

Parts Used

> **Root:** The roots of echinacea are the most valued part for medicinal purposes. They are harvested in the fall or spring when the plant's energy is concentrated in the roots. Echinacea root contains beneficial compounds such as alkamides, polysaccharides, and glycoproteins.

> **Aerial Parts:** The above-ground parts of echinacea, including the flowers, leaves, and stems, are also used in herbal preparations. They contain essential oils, flavonoids, and other bioactive compounds.

Cultivation

Echinacea is perennial and relatively easy to grow, thriving in sunny locations with well-draining soil. Here are key cultivation tips:

- ➢ **Light:** Echinacea prefers full sun to partial shade. Ensure plants receive at least 6 hours of direct sunlight daily for optimal growth and flower production.
- ➢ **Soil:** Use well-draining soil with a slightly alkaline to neutral pH (around 6.0 to 7.0). Sandy loam or loamy soil enriched with organic matter is ideal.
- ➢ **Watering:** Water echinacea regularly during its first growing season to establish a deep root system. Once established, it is drought-tolerant and requires minimal watering.
- ➢ **Propagation:** Echinacea can be propagated from seeds or by dividing existing plants. Directly sow seeds in the garden in early spring or start seeds indoors 6-8 weeks before the last frost date.

Properties

- ➢ **Immune-Stimulating:** Echinacea enhances immune function by increasing the production and activity of white blood cells, particularly during infections such as colds and flu.
- ➢ **Anti-inflammatory:** The herb exhibits anti-inflammatory properties, reducing inflammation and promoting healing in conditions such as arthritis and skin irritations.
- ➢ **Antioxidant:** Echinacea is rich in antioxidants, such as flavonoids and caffeic acid derivatives, which help neutralize free radicals and protect cells from oxidative damage.
- ➢ **Antiviral and Antibacterial:** Echinacea has antiviral and antibacterial properties that inhibit the growth of pathogens and support overall immune health.

Uses

- ➢ **Immune Support:** Echinacea is widely used to prevent and treat common colds, flu, and upper respiratory infections. It helps reduce the severity and duration of symptoms.
- ➢ **Wound Healing:** Applied topically, echinacea accelerates wound healing and reduces inflammation. It is used for minor cuts, burns, insect bites, and skin irritations.
- ➢ **Digestive Health:** Echinacea root is beneficial for promoting digestive health, relieving gastrointestinal discomfort, and supporting overall gut function.
- ➢ **Overall Wellness:** Regular use of echinacea promotes overall

wellness by strengthening the immune system and enhancing resilience to infections and stress.

Echinacea's robust immune-boosting properties and versatile applications make it a valuable addition to both traditional herbal medicine and modern wellness practices. Whether used preventatively to bolster immune defenses or therapeutically to address acute health concerns, echinacea continues to captivate with its potent benefits and natural healing capabilities.

Plant Profile: Lavender

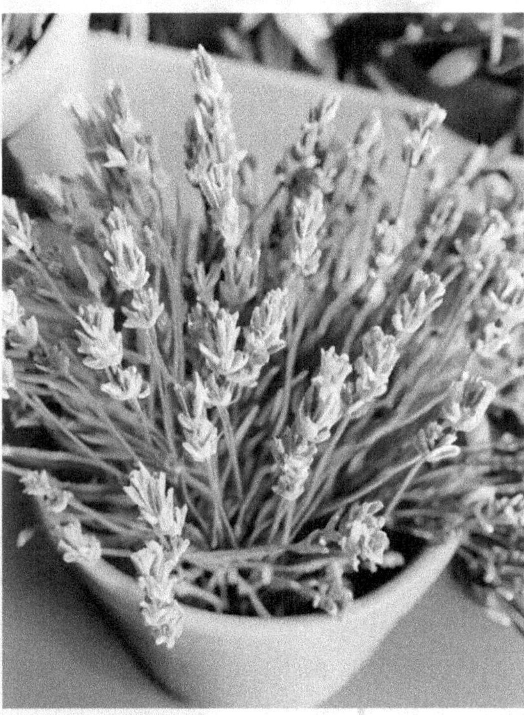

Lavender, cherished for its soothing aroma and versatile medicinal properties, belongs to the genus Lavandula within the Lamiaceae family. In this profile, we explore the identification, parts used, cultivation, properties, and diverse uses of lavender, highlighting its role as a cornerstone of herbal medicine and aromatherapy.

Identification

➢ **Appearance:** Lavender is characterized by slender, woody stems adorned with linear or lance-shaped leaves that are gray-green in color and highly aromatic when crushed. The plant forms compact, bushy shrubs with spikes of small, fragrant flowers arranged in terminal clusters.

➢ **Flowers:** Lavender flowers are tubular and range in color from pale purple to deep violet-blue, attracting pollinators such as bees and butterflies during the blooming season.

Parts Used

➢ **Flowers:** The flowers of lavender are the primary part used for medicinal and aromatic purposes. They are harvested when in full bloom to capture their essential oils and beneficial compounds.

➢ **Essential Oil:** Lavender essential oil is extracted from the flowers through steam distillation. It contains active compounds including linalool, linalyl acetate, and terpenes, which contribute to its therapeutic properties.

Cultivation

Lavender is a perennial herb known for its resilience and adaptability. Here are key cultivation tips:

- **Light:** Lavender thrives in full sun, requiring at least 6-8 hours of direct sunlight daily for optimal growth and flower production.
- **Soil:** Use well-draining, sandy or rocky soil with a slightly alkaline to neutral pH (around 6.5 to 7.5). Good drainage is essential to prevent root rot.
- **Watering:** Lavender is drought-tolerant once established. Water deeply but infrequently, allowing the soil to dry out between waterings to mimic its native Mediterranean habitat.
- **Pruning:** Regular pruning after flowering helps maintain plant shape, encourages new growth, and prolongs the life of the plant.

Properties

- **Sedative:** Lavender exerts a calming and sedative effect on the nervous system, making it effective for reducing anxiety, stress, and promoting relaxation.
- **Antimicrobial:** The essential oil of lavender possesses antimicrobial properties, inhibiting the growth of bacteria and fungi. It is used topically to cleanse wounds and prevent infections.
- **Anti-inflammatory:** Lavender helps reduce inflammation and soothe skin irritations, making it valuable for treating minor burns, insect bites, and dermatitis.
- **Antioxidant:** Rich in antioxidants, lavender helps neutralize free radicals, protecting cells from oxidative stress and supporting overall skin health.

Uses

- **Aromatherapy:** Lavender essential oil is widely used in aromatherapy to promote relaxation, improve sleep quality, and alleviate symptoms of anxiety and depression.
- **Topical Applications:** Infused lavender oils, balms, and creams are applied topically to soothe skin irritations, sunburns, cuts, and bruises.
- **Culinary:** Culinary lavender flowers are used sparingly to flavor desserts, beverages, and savory dishes, adding a floral and aromatic touch.
- **Household:** Lavender sachets and potpourris are used to freshen linens, closets, and

rooms, imparting a pleasant scent while repelling moths and insects.

Lavender's exquisite fragrance and therapeutic benefits have made it a beloved herb across cultures and centuries. Whether enjoyed for its calming aroma, medicinal properties, or culinary delights, lavender continues to captivate with its myriad uses and profound impact on health and well-being.

Lavender stands as a testament to nature's ability to nurture and heal, offering a symphony of scent and therapeutic benefits. As you embrace lavender in your herbal journey, may its calming influence and versatile applications enrich your daily life and promote holistic wellness. Embrace the legacy of lavender, a plant that bridges ancient herbal wisdom with modern health practices, and discover the profound impact of its gentle yet potent healing touch.

Plant Profile: Peppermint

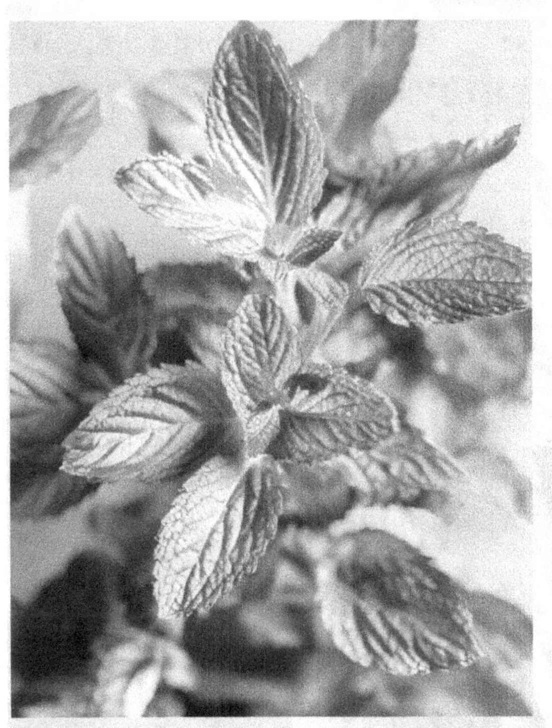

Peppermint, celebrated for its refreshing aroma and therapeutic properties, belongs to the Mentha genus within the Lamiaceae family. In this profile, we explore the identification, parts used, cultivation, properties, and diverse uses of peppermint, highlighting its significance in both culinary delights and herbal medicine.

Identification

> Appearance: Peppermint is a perennial herb with square stems that grow upright, reaching heights of 12-36 inches (30-90 cm). The leaves are dark green with reddish veins, lance-shaped, and serrated along the edges. When crushed, the leaves emit a strong, refreshing minty aroma.

> Flowers: Peppermint produces spikes of small, purple to pinkish flowers in late spring to summer. These flowers attract bees and other pollinators.

Parts Used

- **Leaves:** The leaves of peppermint are the primary part used for medicinal and culinary purposes. They are harvested before flowering for optimal flavor and potency.
- **Essential Oil:** Peppermint essential oil is extracted from the leaves and flowering tops through steam distillation. It contains menthol, menthone, and other volatile compounds that contribute to its distinctive aroma and therapeutic effects.

Cultivation

Peppermint is known for its vigorous growth and adaptability. Here are key cultivation tips:

- **Light:** Peppermint thrives in full sun to partial shade. Ensure plants receive at least 4-6 hours of direct sunlight daily for robust growth.
- **Soil:** Use moist, well-draining soil with a pH between 6.0 and 7.5. Peppermint can tolerate a range of soil types but prefers loamy soil rich in organic matter.
- **Watering:** Keep the soil consistently moist but not waterlogged. Water deeply when the top inch of soil feels dry, especially during hot weather.
- **Propagation:** Peppermint is propagated through division of existing plants or by taking stem cuttings. Plant cuttings in moist soil or water until roots develop, then transplant into the garden or larger pots.

Properties

- **Digestive Aid:** Peppermint is known for its carminative properties, soothing digestive discomfort such as bloating, gas, and indigestion.
- **Antispasmodic:** The menthol in peppermint relaxes smooth muscles, relieving muscle spasms and cramps, including those in the digestive tract.
- **Antimicrobial:** Peppermint has antimicrobial properties that inhibit the growth of bacteria and fungi, contributing to oral health and wound care.
- **Menthol Cooling Effect:** Menthol provides a cooling sensation that alleviates itching, inflammation, and discomfort associated with skin conditions and minor injuries.

Uses

- **Digestive Health:** Peppermint tea is consumed to ease digestive issues, reduce nausea, and promote healthy digestion after meals.
- **Oral Care:** Peppermint oil is added to toothpaste, mouthwashes, and oral care

products for its antibacterial properties and refreshing taste.

➤ Topical Applications: Peppermint essential oil is diluted and applied topically to relieve headaches, muscle soreness, and joint pain through massage or as a compress.

➤ Culinary Delights: Fresh or dried peppermint leaves are used to flavor teas, desserts, salads, and savory dishes, adding a refreshing minty taste.

Peppermint's invigorating aroma and therapeutic benefits have made it a cherished herb throughout history. Whether enjoyed for its culinary zest, digestive support, or topical relief, peppermint continues to captivate with its versatility and effectiveness in promoting health and well-being.

Plant Profile: Rosemary

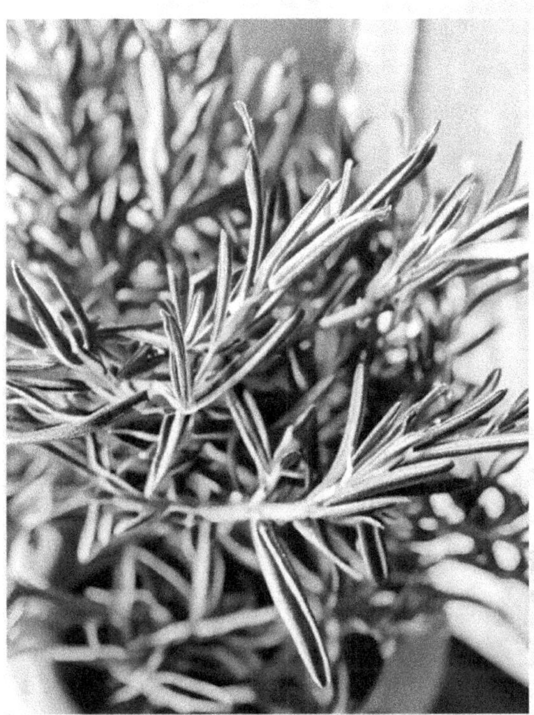

Rosemary, esteemed for its robust flavor and medicinal properties, belongs to the genus Salvia within the Lamiaceae family. In this profile, we explore the identification, parts used, cultivation, properties, and diverse uses of rosemary, highlighting its versatility in culinary arts and therapeutic applications.

Identification

➤ Appearance: Rosemary is an evergreen shrub with woody stems that can grow upright or trail along the ground. The needle-like leaves are narrow, aromatic, and dark green on top with a silvery underside. They are arranged oppositely on the stem and release a pine-like fragrance when crushed.

➤ Flowers: Rosemary produces small, tubular flowers that range in color from white to pale blue, clustered along the stem tips. The flowers attract bees and other pollinators during the blooming season.

Parts Used

➤ Leaves: The leaves of rosemary are the primary part used for culinary and medicinal purposes. They are harvested throughout the year but are most flavorful just before the plant blooms.

➢ **Essential Oil:** Rosemary essential oil is extracted from the leaves and flowering tops through steam distillation. It contains cineole, camphor, and other volatile compounds that contribute to its aroma and therapeutic effects.

Cultivation

Rosemary thrives in warm, Mediterranean-like climates but can be grown in various regions with proper care. Here are key cultivation tips:

➢ **Light:** Rosemary requires full sun to thrive. Plant it in a location that receives at least 6-8 hours of direct sunlight daily.

➢ **Soil:** Use well-draining, sandy or loamy soil with a pH between 6.0 and 7.0. Rosemary is tolerant of poor soils but prefers soil that is not overly rich or water-retentive.

➢ **Watering:** Water rosemary deeply but infrequently, allowing the soil to dry out between waterings. It is drought-tolerant once established and prefers slightly dry conditions.

➢ **Propagation:** Rosemary can be propagated from seeds, cuttings, or layering. Take stem cuttings from healthy plants and root them in well-draining soil or water until roots develop.

Properties

➢ **Antioxidant:** Rosemary contains antioxidants such as rosmarinic acid and carnosic acid, which help neutralize free radicals and protect cells from oxidative stress.

➢ **Anti-inflammatory:** The anti-inflammatory properties of rosemary make it beneficial for reducing inflammation in joints, muscles, and tissues.

➢ **Cognitive Function:** Rosemary is known to enhance memory, concentration, and cognitive function. It is often used in aromatherapy to promote mental clarity and alertness.

➢ **Antimicrobial:** Rosemary exhibits antimicrobial properties that inhibit the growth of bacteria and fungi, supporting oral health and wound healing.

Uses

➢ **Culinary:** Fresh or dried rosemary leaves are used to flavor a variety of dishes, including meats, vegetables, breads, and soups. It adds a robust, pine-like flavor.

➢ **Aromatherapy:** Rosemary essential oil is used in aromatherapy to improve mental focus, alleviate stress, and enhance mood. It can be diffused, inhaled directly, or added to massage oils.

➢ **Hair and Skin Care:** Rosemary infused oils or rinses are applied topically to stimulate hair growth, improve scalp health, and enhance skin tone. It is used in shampoos, conditioners, and skincare products.

➢ **Medicinal Teas:** Rosemary leaves can be steeped in hot water to create an herbal tea that aids digestion, relieves headaches, and supports overall wellness.

Rosemary's robust flavor and therapeutic benefits have made it a cherished herb across cultures and centuries. Whether used to elevate culinary creations, promote mental clarity, or enhance hair and skin health, rosemary continues to captivate with its aromatic essence and profound impact on well-being.

Plant Profile: Turmeric

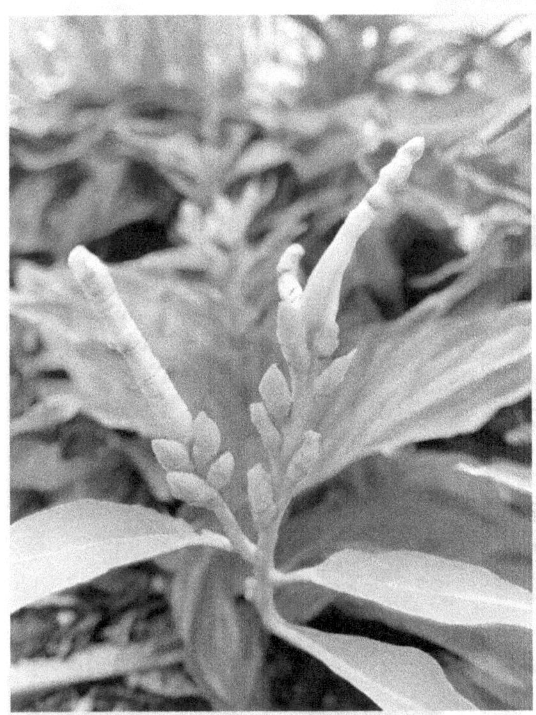

Turmeric, revered for its vibrant color and potent medicinal properties, belongs to the Curcuma genus within the Zingiberaceae family. In this profile, we explore the identification, parts used, cultivation, properties, and diverse uses of turmeric, highlighting its significance in both culinary traditions and herbal medicine.

Identification

➢ **Appearance:** Turmeric is a perennial herbaceous plant that grows up to 3 feet (1 meter) tall. It features long, lance-shaped leaves that arise from a central rhizome. The rhizome, which is the part harvested for use, is bright orange-yellow inside and covered with a brownish skin.

➢ **Flowers:** Turmeric produces spikes of small, yellowish-white flowers that emerge from the base of the leaves. However, the flowers are rarely the focus due to the primary use of the rhizome.

Parts Used

- ➤ **Rhizome:** The rhizome of turmeric is the primary part used for its culinary and medicinal benefits. It is harvested, cleaned, boiled, dried, and then ground into a fine powder known as turmeric spice. Fresh turmeric rhizomes can also be used grated or sliced in cooking.
- ➤ **Curcumin:** Curcumin is the active compound found in turmeric responsible for its vibrant yellow color and many of its health benefits. It has potent antioxidant, anti-inflammatory, and antimicrobial properties.

Cultivation

Turmeric is native to South Asia and thrives in warm, humid climates. Here are key cultivation tips:

- ➤ **Climate:** Turmeric prefers temperatures between 68-86°F (20-30°C) and high humidity. It can be grown outdoors in tropical and subtropical regions or indoors in pots in cooler climates.
- ➤ **Soil:** Use rich, well-draining soil with a pH of 6.0-7.8. Sandy loam or loamy soil enriched with organic matter is ideal for promoting rhizome growth.
- ➤ **Watering:** Keep the soil consistently moist but not waterlogged. Turmeric requires regular watering, especially during the growing season, but reduce watering during dormancy.
- ➤ **Propagation:** Turmeric is propagated from rhizome pieces with at least one viable bud. Plant rhizome pieces in shallow furrows or containers with the buds facing upward.

Properties

- ➤ **Anti-inflammatory:** Turmeric is renowned for its anti-inflammatory properties, attributed to curcumin, which helps reduce inflammation in joints, muscles, and tissues.
- ➤ **Antioxidant:** Curcumin acts as a powerful antioxidant, scavenging free radicals and protecting cells from oxidative stress. It supports overall cellular health and longevity.
- ➤ **Digestive Aid:** Turmeric promotes digestive health by stimulating bile production, aiding in fat digestion, and reducing symptoms of bloating and gas.
- ➤ **Antimicrobial:** Turmeric exhibits antimicrobial properties that inhibit the growth of bacteria, fungi, and viruses, contributing to immune support and wound healing.

Uses

- ➤ **Culinary:** Turmeric is a staple spice in South Asian cuisine, imparting a bright yellow color and warm, slightly bitter flavor to dishes such as curries, rice, soups, and stews.

➢ **Medicinal Teas:** Turmeric tea or golden milk, made with turmeric powder or grated fresh turmeric, is consumed for its anti-inflammatory and immune-boosting benefits.

➢ **Topical Applications:** Turmeric paste or oil is applied topically to soothe skin irritations, reduce acne inflammation, and promote wound healing.

➢ **Supplements:** Turmeric supplements, often standardized for curcumin content, are used to support joint health, reduce inflammation, and promote overall well-being.

Turmeric's rich cultural heritage and therapeutic benefits have made it a valued herb worldwide. Whether used to enhance culinary creations, support digestive health, or alleviate inflammation, turmeric continues to captivate with its vibrant hue and profound impact on health and wellness.

Plant Profile: Valerian

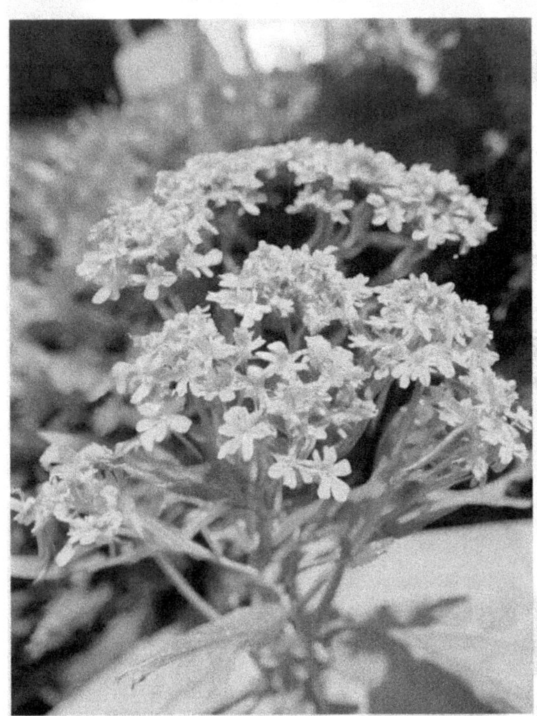

Valerian, renowned for its sedative and calming properties, belongs to the Valeriana genus within the Caprifoliaceae family. In this profile, we explore the identification, parts used, cultivation, properties, and diverse uses of valerian, highlighting its role as a valuable herb in promoting relaxation and sleep.

Identification

➢ **Appearance:** Valerian is a perennial herbaceous plant that grows up to 5 feet (1.5 meters) tall. It features hollow, grooved stems with pairs of opposite, fern-like leaves that are deeply divided into toothed segments. The plant bears clusters of small, fragrant white to pinkish flowers in summer.

➢ **Root:** The root of valerian is the main part used for

medicinal purposes. It is thick, gnarled, and has a distinct, earthy odor when dried.

Parts Used

> **Root:** The underground root of valerian is harvested for its medicinal compounds, including volatile oils (valerenic acid), valepotriates, and alkaloids. It is collected in the autumn of the plant's second year or later for optimal potency.

Cultivation

Valerian is native to Europe and Asia but is cultivated worldwide for its medicinal benefits. Here are key cultivation tips:

> **Climate:** Valerian thrives in temperate climates with cool summers. It prefers rich, loamy soil with good drainage and can tolerate partial shade.

> **Propagation:** Valerian is propagated from seed or by dividing established plants. Sow seeds in the spring or fall, and space plants 12-18 inches (30-45 cm) apart.

> **Watering:** Keep the soil consistently moist, especially during dry spells, but avoid waterlogged conditions, which can lead to root rot.

> **Maintenance:** Cut back flowering stems to promote root growth and prevent self-seeding, as valerian can become invasive.

Properties

> **Sedative:** Valerian is primarily known for its sedative and calming effects on the nervous system. It enhances the activity of gamma-aminobutyric acid (GABA), a neurotransmitter that helps regulate anxiety and sleep.

> **Anxiolytic:** Valerian has mild anxiolytic properties, reducing feelings of anxiety and promoting relaxation without causing drowsiness during the day.

> **Muscle Relaxant:** The herb acts as a muscle relaxant, easing tension and spasms in the muscles, making it beneficial for conditions like menstrual cramps and muscle pain.

> **Hypnotic:** Valerian improves sleep quality by shortening the time it takes to fall asleep and enhancing deep sleep phases. It is used to treat insomnia and sleep disorders.

Uses

> **Sleep Aid:** Valerian root is commonly used as a natural remedy for insomnia and improving sleep quality. It is often brewed into teas, tinctures, or taken as capsules before bedtime.

- ➢ Anxiety Relief: Valerian extracts or supplements are used to alleviate symptoms of anxiety, nervousness, and stress-related disorders.
- ➢ Digestive Aid: Valerian can be used to relieve digestive spasms, cramps, and discomfort associated with nervous tension.
- ➢ Topical Applications: Valerian oil or extracts are sometimes applied topically to alleviate muscle pain, tension headaches, and minor skin irritations.

Valerian's gentle yet effective sedative properties have made it a popular choice in herbal medicine for centuries. Whether used to promote restful sleep, reduce anxiety, or soothe muscle tension, valerian continues to offer natural support for holistic well-being.

Plant Profile: Ginger

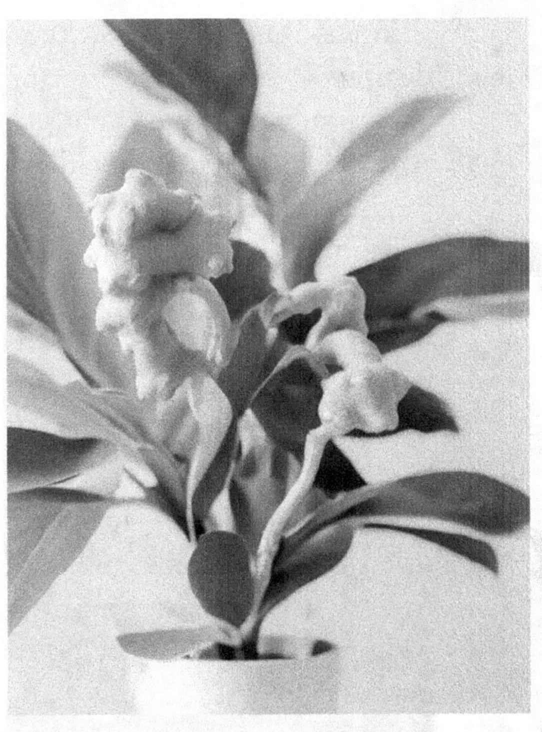

Ginger, prized for its pungent aroma and myriad health benefits, belongs to the Zingiberaceae family. In this profile, we delve into the identification, parts used, cultivation, properties, and diverse uses of ginger, highlighting its versatility in both culinary delights and herbal medicine.

Identification

- ➢ Appearance: Ginger is a perennial herbaceous plant with thick, knobby rhizomes that grow underground. The above-ground stems, known as pseudostems, can reach heights of 2-4 feet (60-120 cm). The leaves are long, narrow, and green with a prominent midrib.
- ➢ Rhizome: The rhizome of ginger is the primary part used for its culinary and medicinal properties. It is harvested when mature, washed, and dried before use. Fresh ginger rhizomes are also grated, sliced, or juiced for immediate consumption.

Parts Used

- ➤ **Rhizome:** Ginger rhizome is rich in bioactive compounds such as gingerol, shogaol, and zingerone, which impart its characteristic flavor and medicinal properties. It can be used fresh, dried, powdered, or as an essential oil.

Cultivation

Ginger is native to Southeast Asia but is now cultivated in tropical and subtropical regions worldwide. Here are key cultivation tips:

- ➤ **Climate:** Ginger thrives in warm, humid climates with temperatures between 75-85°F (24-29°C). It requires partial shade and protection from direct sunlight.
- ➤ **Soil:** Plant ginger in well-draining, loamy soil enriched with organic matter. The soil pH should ideally be between 5.5 and 6.5.
- ➤ **Watering:** Keep the soil consistently moist but not waterlogged. Ginger requires regular watering, especially during dry periods, but reduce watering during dormancy.
- ➤ **Propagation:** Ginger is propagated from rhizome divisions. Choose healthy, plump rhizomes with visible buds (eyes) for planting.

Properties

- ➤ **Anti-inflammatory:** Ginger exhibits potent anti-inflammatory properties, reducing inflammation in joints, muscles, and tissues. It is beneficial for arthritis and other inflammatory conditions.
- ➤ **Digestive Aid:** Ginger stimulates digestion by promoting the production of digestive enzymes and bile. It helps relieve nausea, indigestion, and gastrointestinal discomfort.
- ➤ **Antiemetic:** Ginger is effective in alleviating nausea and vomiting, including motion sickness, morning sickness during pregnancy, and chemotherapy-induced nausea.
- ➤ **Antioxidant:** The antioxidants in ginger, such as gingerol and zingerone, help neutralize free radicals, protecting cells from oxidative stress and promoting overall health.

Uses

- ➤ **Culinary Delights:** Fresh or dried ginger rhizomes are used to add flavor and aroma to a wide range of dishes, including curries, stir-fries, soups, and marinades.
- ➤ **Digestive Health:** Ginger tea or ginger-infused water is consumed to ease digestive discomfort, reduce bloating, and improve overall gut health.
- ➤ **Natural Remedies:** Ginger is used in traditional medicine to

treat colds, flu, headaches, and menstrual cramps. It can be brewed into teas, tinctures, or taken as capsules.

➤ Topical Applications: Ginger oil or poultices are applied topically to relieve muscle pain, joint stiffness, and headaches through massage or compresses.

Ginger's distinctive flavor and therapeutic benefits have made it a staple in both kitchens and medicine cabinets worldwide. Whether enjoyed for its culinary zest, digestive support, or natural healing properties, ginger continues to captivate with its versatility and effectiveness in promoting health and well-being.

Plant Profile: Calendula

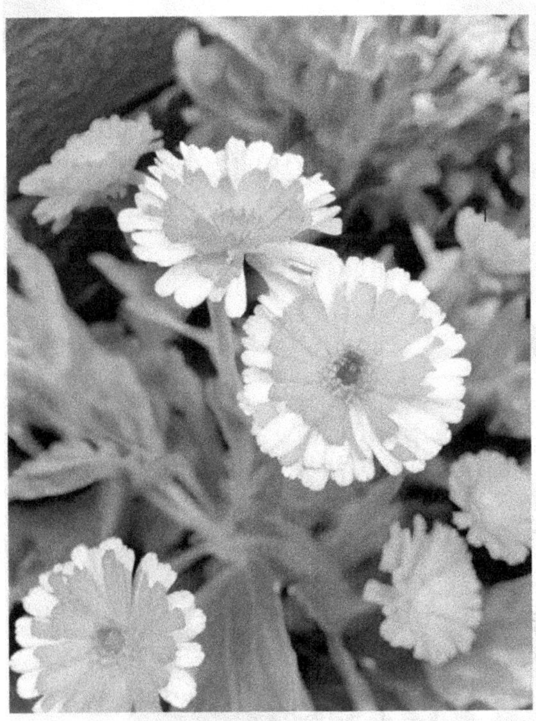

Calendula, esteemed for its vibrant flowers and medicinal properties, belongs to the genus Calendula within the Asteraceae family. In this profile, we explore the identification, parts used, cultivation, properties, and diverse uses of calendula, highlighting its versatility in both skincare and herbal medicine.

Identification

➤ Appearance: Calendula, also known as pot marigold, is an annual or perennial herbaceous plant. It features bright yellow to orange flowers with a daisy-like appearance, growing on sturdy stems. The leaves are lance-shaped, green, and slightly hairy.

➤ Flowers: The vibrant calendula flowers bloom profusely from spring through fall, attracting pollinators such as bees and butterflies. They are harvested when fully open for their medicinal properties.

Parts Used

➤ Flowers: Calendula flowers are the primary part used for medicinal and skincare purposes. They are harvested at full bloom and can be used fresh or dried.

➤ Extracts/Oils: Calendula extracts, oils, and infusions are prepared from the flowers to capture their beneficial compounds, including flavonoids, saponins, and carotenoids.

Cultivation

Calendula is native to Mediterranean regions but is now cultivated worldwide for its ornamental beauty and medicinal benefits. Here are key cultivation tips:

- ➢ Climate: Calendula thrives in cool to moderate climates and can tolerate frost. It prefers full sun but can also grow in partial shade.
- ➢ Soil: Plant calendula in well-draining soil enriched with organic matter. It tolerates various soil types but thrives in loamy, fertile soil.
- ➢ Watering: Keep the soil consistently moist but not waterlogged. Water calendula plants deeply during dry spells and avoid overhead watering to prevent fungal diseases.
- ➢ Propagation: Calendula is easily grown from seeds sown directly into the garden bed in spring or fall. Thin seedlings to allow proper spacing for growth.

Properties

- ➢ Anti-inflammatory: Calendula has powerful anti-inflammatory properties, making it effective for soothing skin irritations, rashes, and minor wounds.
- ➢ Antimicrobial: The antimicrobial actions of calendula help prevent infections and promote healing of cuts, scrapes, and burns.
- ➢ Antioxidant: Rich in antioxidants like flavonoids and carotenoids, calendula protects the skin from free radical damage and supports overall skin health.
- ➢ Emollient: Calendula is emollient, meaning it moisturizes and softens the skin, making it beneficial for dry, chapped skin and lips.

Uses

- ➢ Skincare: Calendula-infused oils, creams, and salves are applied topically to soothe eczema, dermatitis, sunburns, and diaper rash.
- ➢ Wound Healing: Calendula extracts are used in wound dressings and ointments to promote faster healing of cuts, bruises, and minor burns.
- ➢ Oral Care: Calendula mouthwashes and rinses are used to support oral health, reduce inflammation of gums, and alleviate mouth ulcers.
- ➢ Internal Use: Calendula tea or tincture is consumed internally to support digestion, reduce inflammation in the digestive

tract, and boost the immune system.

Calendula's gentle yet potent healing properties have made it a cherished herb in both traditional and modern herbal medicine. Whether used for its skin-soothing effects, wound healing properties, or digestive support, calendula continues to captivate with its versatility and effectiveness in promoting health and well-being.

Plant Profile: Lemon Balm

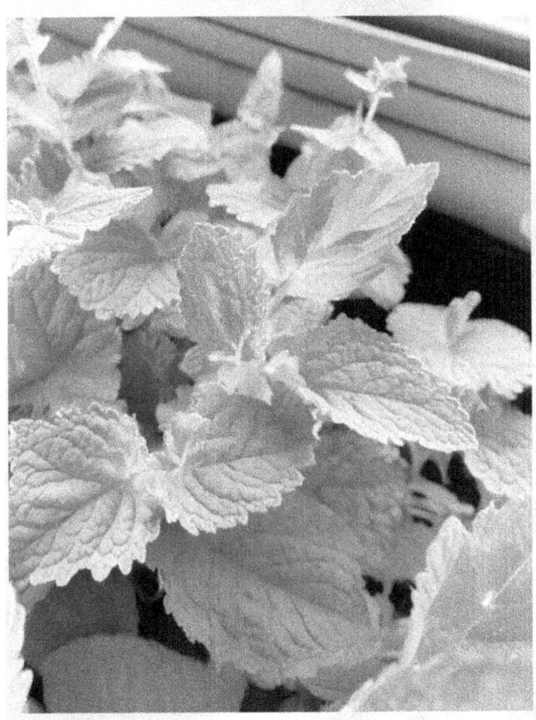

Lemon Balm, revered for its citrusy fragrance and medicinal properties, belongs to the genus Melissa within the Lamiaceae family. In this profile, we explore the identification, parts used, cultivation, properties, and diverse uses of lemon balm, highlighting its versatility in both culinary delights and herbal medicine.

Identification

> **Appearance:** Lemon balm is a perennial herbaceous plant with square stems that grow upright to about 2 feet (60 cm) tall. The leaves are heart-shaped, deeply veined, and emit a strong lemon scent when crushed. Small clusters of white or pale yellow flowers appear in summer.

> **Fragrance:** The leaves of lemon balm release a distinct lemony aroma due to their high content of essential oils, primarily citronellal and citral.

Parts Used

> **Leaves:** The leaves of lemon balm are the primary part used for their medicinal and culinary benefits. They are harvested before flowering for optimal flavor and potency.

> **Essential Oil:** Lemon balm essential oil is extracted from the leaves and flowering tops through steam distillation. It contains citronellal, citral, and other volatile compounds that contribute to its aromatic and therapeutic effects.

Cultivation

Lemon balm is native to the Mediterranean region but is now cultivated worldwide for its aromatic leaves and medicinal properties. Here are key cultivation tips:

- **Climate:** Lemon balm thrives in temperate climates with moderate temperatures and full sun to partial shade. It can tolerate a range of soil types but prefers well-draining, fertile soil.
- **Propagation:** Lemon balm is propagated from seeds, cuttings, or division of mature plants. Seeds should be sown indoors in early spring or directly in the garden after the last frost.
- **Watering:** Keep the soil consistently moist but not waterlogged. Water deeply during dry spells and mulch around plants to retain moisture.
- **Maintenance:** Trim lemon balm regularly to encourage bushy growth and prevent it from becoming invasive. Divide plants every few years to rejuvenate growth and maintain vigor.

Properties

- **Sedative:** Lemon balm has mild sedative properties that promote relaxation and ease nervous tension. It is beneficial for reducing anxiety, stress, and promoting restful sleep.
- **Antioxidant:** The antioxidants in lemon balm, including rosmarinic acid and flavonoids, help neutralize free radicals and protect cells from oxidative damage.
- **Antimicrobial:** Lemon balm exhibits antimicrobial properties that inhibit the growth of bacteria and fungi, supporting immune health and wound healing.
- **Digestive Aid:** Lemon balm aids digestion by stimulating bile production and soothing gastrointestinal spasms and discomfort.

Uses

- **Herbal Teas:** Lemon balm leaves are infused in hot water to create a soothing herbal tea that promotes relaxation, reduces stress, and aids digestion.
- **Culinary:** Fresh or dried lemon balm leaves are used as a culinary herb to flavor salads, soups, sauces, and desserts. It adds a subtle lemony flavor.
- **Topical Applications:** Lemon balm salves, creams, or infused oils are applied topically to soothe insect bites, minor skin irritations, and herpes cold sores.
- **Aromatherapy:** Lemon balm essential oil is diffused or inhaled directly to uplift

mood, improve concentration, and alleviate symptoms of anxiety.

Lemon balm's gentle yet effective medicinal properties have made it a beloved herb for centuries. Whether enjoyed in teas, culinary dishes, or aromatherapy, lemon balm continues to captivate with its refreshing aroma and therapeutic benefits.

Plant Profile: Dandelion

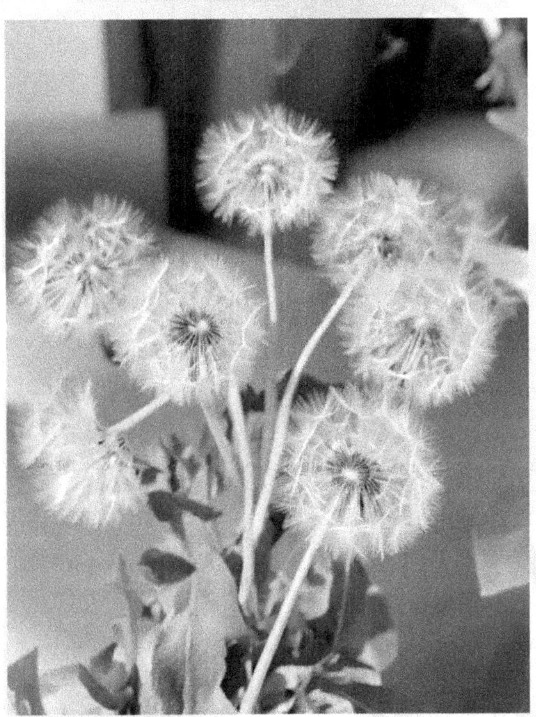

Dandelion, often considered a humble weed, holds profound medicinal properties and culinary uses, belonging to the genus Taraxacum within the Asteraceae family. In this profile, we explore the identification, parts used, cultivation, properties, and diverse uses of dandelion, highlighting its versatility and nutritional richness.

Identification

> Appearance: Dandelion is a perennial herbaceous plant with deeply toothed, basal leaves that form a rosette close to the ground. The leaves can grow up to 12 inches (30 cm) long and emit a milky sap when broken. Yellow, solitary flower heads rise on hollow stems, maturing into spherical seed heads (puffballs) with feathery seeds.

> Flowers: The bright yellow dandelion flowers bloom from early spring through late fall, attracting pollinators such as bees. Each flower head matures into a round seed head that releases parachuted seeds when blown by the wind.

Parts Used

> Leaves: Dandelion leaves are harvested before the plant flowers for optimal tenderness and flavor. They are rich in vitamins (A, C, K), minerals (iron, calcium, potassium), and antioxidants (beta-carotene, lutein).

> Root: Dandelion roots are harvested in early spring or late fall when the plant is dormant. They are long, tapering, and deep-reaching,

containing bitter principles (taraxacin and taraxacerin) that support digestive health.

➤ Flowers: Dandelion flowers can be harvested and used fresh or dried for their mild sweetness and bright color in culinary preparations.

Cultivation

Dandelion is native to Europe and Asia but has naturalized throughout temperate regions worldwide. Here are key cultivation tips:

➤ Soil: Dandelions thrive in well-draining, fertile soil but can tolerate poor soil conditions. They prefer neutral to slightly acidic pH levels.

➤ Sunlight: Plant dandelions in full sun to partial shade. They are adaptable and grow well in both open fields and lawns.

➤ Propagation: Dandelions propagate through wind-dispersed seeds and can self-seed prolifically. They also reproduce through deep taproots that can be divided and replanted.

➤ Maintenance: Control dandelion growth by regular mowing or harvesting. Harvest leaves before they become bitter and tough.

Properties

➤ Diuretic: Dandelion acts as a gentle diuretic, promoting urine production and helping flush excess fluids and toxins from the body. It supports kidney health and reduces bloating.

➤ Digestive Aid: Dandelion stimulates appetite, enhances bile production, and aids digestion. It is used to relieve constipation, indigestion, and liver congestion.

➤ Anti-inflammatory: Dandelion exhibits anti-inflammatory properties that help reduce inflammation in joints and tissues. It is beneficial for conditions like arthritis and gout.

➤ Antioxidant: The antioxidants in dandelion, including beta-carotene and polyphenols, protect cells from oxidative stress and support overall health.

Uses

➤ Culinary: Dandelion leaves are used fresh in salads, sautéed as greens, or brewed into teas. The flowers are used to make dandelion wine or infused into syrups and jellies.

➤ Medicinal Teas: Dandelion leaf tea or root tea is consumed to support liver detoxification, promote digestion, and cleanse the urinary tract.

➤ Herbal Remedies: Dandelion extracts or tinctures are used in herbal medicine to treat digestive disorders, skin conditions, and support kidney function.

➤ **Cosmetic Uses:** Dandelion extract is used in skincare products for its antioxidant properties, promoting youthful skin and reducing inflammation.

Dandelion's nutritional richness and therapeutic benefits have made it a valued herb for centuries. Whether enjoyed for its culinary versatility, medicinal properties, or ecological benefits, dandelion continues to captivate with its resilience and holistic wellness support.

Plant Profile: Sage

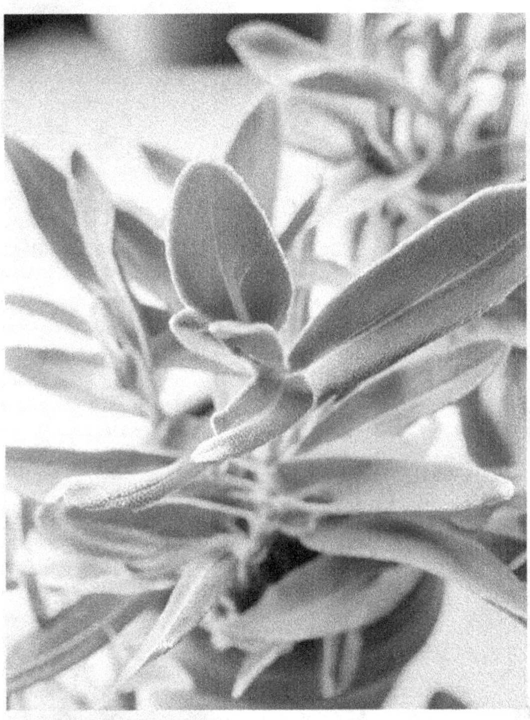

Sage, esteemed for its aromatic foliage and medicinal properties, belongs to the genus Salvia within the Lamiaceae family. In this profile, we explore the identification, parts used, cultivation, properties, and diverse uses of sage, highlighting its versatility in both culinary delights and herbal medicine.

Identification

➤ **Appearance:** Sage is a perennial woody shrub with gray-green, oval-shaped leaves that are densely covered with fine hairs. The leaves have a distinctive wrinkled texture and are arranged oppositely on square stems. Sage produces small, tubular flowers that range in color from blue and purple to white, depending on the variety.

➤ **Fragrance:** The leaves of sage emit a strong, earthy aroma when crushed, owing to their high concentration of essential oils.

Parts Used

➤ **Leaves:** Sage leaves are the primary part used for culinary and medicinal purposes. They are harvested before flowering for optimal flavor and potency. Fresh leaves are used immediately, while dried leaves are stored for long-term use.

➢ **Essential Oil:** Sage essential oil is extracted from the leaves through steam distillation. It contains potent aromatic compounds such as thujone, camphor, and cineole, which contribute to its therapeutic properties.

Cultivation

Sage is native to the Mediterranean region but is cultivated worldwide for its culinary and medicinal benefits. Here are key cultivation tips:

➢ **Climate:** Sage thrives in full sun and well-draining, sandy soil. It is drought-tolerant once established but benefits from regular watering during dry spells.

➢ **Propagation:** Sage is propagated from seeds, cuttings, or division of established plants. Sow seeds indoors in early spring or directly in the garden after the last frost.

➢ **Soil:** Plant sage in alkaline to neutral soil with a pH between 6.0 and 7.0. Improve soil drainage by adding organic matter such as compost.

➢ **Maintenance:** Prune sage regularly to promote bushy growth and prevent legginess. Trim flower stalks to encourage leaf production and extend the plant's lifespan.

Properties

➢ **Antimicrobial:** Sage exhibits strong antimicrobial properties, inhibiting the growth of bacteria, fungi, and viruses. It is used to treat sore throats, mouth infections, and skin conditions.

➢ **Anti-inflammatory:** The anti-inflammatory compounds in sage, including rosmarinic acid and flavonoids, help reduce inflammation in joints and tissues. It is beneficial for arthritis and inflammatory conditions.

➢ **Antioxidant:** Sage is rich in antioxidants that neutralize free radicals, protecting cells from oxidative stress and supporting overall health.

➢ **Astringent:** Sage acts as an astringent, tightening and toning tissues. It is used topically to reduce excessive sweating and oily skin.

Uses

➢ **Culinary Delights:** Sage leaves are used fresh or dried to flavor meats, poultry, soups, stews, and stuffing. It adds a savory, slightly peppery flavor to dishes.

➢ **Herbal Teas:** Sage tea is brewed from fresh or dried leaves and consumed to soothe sore throats, improve digestion, and support oral health.

➢ **Medicinal Remedies:** Sage tinctures or extracts are used in herbal medicine to alleviate cold symptoms, menstrual cramps, and digestive disorders.

➤ Topical Applications: Sage-infused oils, creams, or compresses are applied to wounds, insect bites, and minor skin irritations for their antiseptic and healing properties.

Sage's aromatic foliage and potent medicinal benefits have made it a cherished herb throughout history. Whether used for its culinary versatility, therapeutic properties, or aromatic allure, sage continues to captivate with its multifaceted contributions to health and well-being.

Plant Profile: Basil

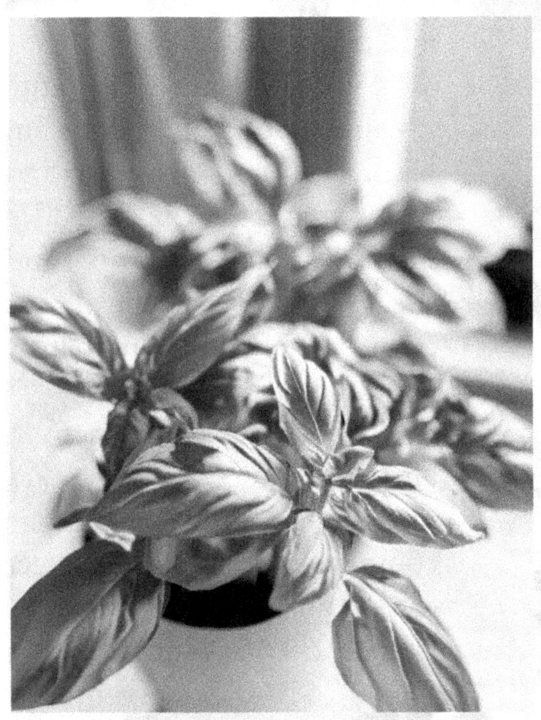

Basil, celebrated for its aromatic leaves and culinary versatility, belongs to the genus Ocimum within the Lamiaceae family. In this profile, we explore the identification, parts used, cultivation, properties, and diverse uses of basil, highlighting its rich cultural history and therapeutic benefits.

Identification

➤ Appearance: Basil is an annual herbaceous plant with tender, green leaves that grow in pairs opposite each other along square stems. The leaves vary in size and shape depending on the variety, ranging from large, smooth leaves to small, serrated ones. Basil plants produce small white or purple flowers arranged in spikes.

➤ Fragrance: Basil leaves emit a strong, sweet, and spicy aroma when crushed, characteristic of its essential oils.

Parts Used

➤ Leaves: Basil leaves are the primary part used for culinary and medicinal purposes. They are harvested throughout the growing season before flowering for optimal flavor and aroma. Fresh leaves are used immediately, while dried leaves are preserved for later use.

➤ **Essential Oil:** Basil essential oil is extracted from the leaves and flowering tops through steam distillation. It contains aromatic compounds such as linalool, eugenol, and methyl chavicol, which contribute to its therapeutic properties.

Cultivation

Basil is native to tropical regions of Asia and Africa but is cultivated worldwide for its culinary significance and medicinal benefits. Here are key cultivation tips:

➤ **Climate:** Basil thrives in warm, sunny conditions with temperatures between 70-90°F (21-32°C). It is sensitive to cold and frost, making it suitable for growing as an annual in temperate climates.

➤ **Soil:** Plant basil in well-draining, fertile soil with a pH level between 6.0 and 7.5. Amend the soil with organic matter such as compost to improve fertility and moisture retention.

➤ **Watering:** Keep the soil consistently moist but not waterlogged. Water basil plants at the base to prevent fungal diseases and promote healthy root development.

➤ **Propagation:** Basil is propagated from seeds or cuttings. Seeds should be sown indoors in early spring or directly in the garden after the last frost. Cuttings root easily in water or moist soil.

Properties

➤ **Antimicrobial:** Basil exhibits antimicrobial properties that help inhibit the growth of bacteria, fungi, and other pathogens. It is used in natural remedies to treat infections and promote healing.

➤ **Anti-inflammatory:** The anti-inflammatory compounds in basil, including eugenol and rosmarinic acid, help reduce inflammation in joints and tissues. It is beneficial for arthritis and inflammatory conditions.

➤ **Antioxidant:** Basil is rich in antioxidants such as flavonoids and phenolic compounds, which protect cells from oxidative stress and support overall health.

➤ **Digestive Aid:** Basil stimulates appetite, aids digestion, and relieves gas and bloating. It is used to alleviate indigestion and promote gastrointestinal health.

Uses

➤ **Culinary Delights:** Basil leaves are used fresh or dried to flavor a wide range of dishes, including pasta sauces, pesto, salads, soups, and infused oils. It adds a fresh, peppery, and slightly sweet flavor to culinary creations.

> Herbal Teas: Basil tea is brewed from fresh leaves and consumed to promote digestion, reduce stress, and uplift mood. It has a refreshing and soothing effect.

> Medicinal Remedies: Basil extracts or tinctures are used in herbal medicine to relieve coughs, colds, and respiratory infections. It is also used topically to soothe insect bites and minor skin irritations.

> Aromatherapy: Basil essential oil is diffused or used in massage blends to reduce anxiety, improve mental clarity, and alleviate headaches.

Basil's aromatic leaves and versatile culinary uses have made it a beloved herb across cultures and centuries. Whether enjoyed for its flavorful impact in cooking, therapeutic benefits in herbal medicine, or aromatic essence in aromatherapy, basil continues to inspire and enrich culinary and wellness practices.

Plant Profile: Oregano

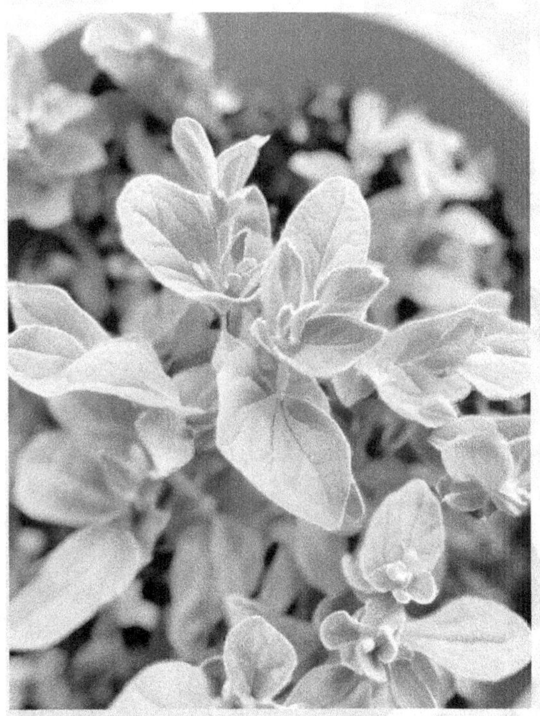

Oregano, prized for its robust flavor and medicinal properties, belongs to the genus Origanum within the Lamiaceae family. In this profile, we delve into the identification, parts used, cultivation, properties, and diverse uses of oregano, highlighting its culinary significance and therapeutic benefits.

Identification

> Appearance: Oregano is a perennial herb with small, oval-shaped leaves that grow in pairs opposite each other on square stems. The leaves are gray-green and covered with fine hairs, giving them a fuzzy texture. Oregano plants produce clusters of small pink or purple flowers that attract pollinators.

- ➤ **Fragrance:** Oregano leaves emit a strong, aromatic scent when crushed, characterized by its essential oils rich in carvacrol, thymol, and limonene.

Parts Used

- ➤ **Leaves:** Oregano leaves are the primary part used for culinary and medicinal purposes. They are harvested throughout the growing season for their intense flavor and aroma. Fresh leaves can be used immediately, while dried leaves retain their potency for long-term storage.
- ➤ **Essential Oil:** Oregano essential oil is extracted from the leaves and flowering tops through steam distillation. It contains potent aromatic compounds that contribute to its therapeutic properties.

Cultivation

Oregano is native to the Mediterranean region but is cultivated worldwide for its culinary appeal and health benefits. Here are key cultivation tips:

- ➤ **Climate:** Oregano thrives in warm, sunny climates with well-draining soil. It is drought-tolerant once established and prefers temperatures between 70-85°F (21-29°C).
- ➤ **Soil:** Plant oregano in sandy, loamy soil with a pH level between 6.0 and 8.0. Amend the soil with organic matter such as compost to improve fertility and drainage.
- ➤ **Watering:** Allow the soil to dry out slightly between waterings. Water oregano at the base to prevent fungal diseases and promote healthy root development.
- ➤ **Propagation:** Oregano is propagated from seeds, cuttings, or division of established plants. Sow seeds indoors in early spring or directly in the garden after the last frost. Cuttings root easily in water or moist soil.

Properties

- ➤ **Antimicrobial:** Oregano exhibits strong antimicrobial properties due to its high content of carvacrol and thymol. It inhibits the growth of bacteria, fungi, and parasites.
- ➤ **Anti-inflammatory:** The anti-inflammatory compounds in oregano, including rosmarinic acid and beta-caryophyllene, help reduce inflammation in the body. It is beneficial for arthritis and digestive disorders.
- ➤ **Antioxidant:** Oregano is rich in antioxidants such as flavonoids and phenolic acids, which protect cells from

oxidative damage caused by free radicals.

➤ **Digestive Aid:** Oregano stimulates digestion, relieves gas and bloating, and supports overall gastrointestinal health.

Uses

➤ **Culinary Delights:** Oregano leaves are used fresh or dried to flavor Mediterranean dishes, including pizzas, pasta sauces, salads, and marinades. It adds a savory, slightly peppery flavor and aroma to culinary creations.

➤ **Herbal Teas:** Oregano tea is brewed from fresh or dried leaves and consumed to alleviate indigestion, promote respiratory health, and boost immunity. It has a warming and soothing effect.

➤ **Medicinal Remedies:** Oregano extracts or tinctures are used in herbal medicine to treat respiratory infections, colds, and sore throats. It is also applied topically to relieve muscle pain and insect bites.

➤ **Aromatherapy:** Oregano essential oil is diffused or used in massage oils to alleviate stress, enhance mental clarity, and support immune function.

Oregano's aromatic leaves and potent health benefits have made it a staple herb in kitchens and apothecaries alike. Whether enjoyed for its culinary versatility, therapeutic properties, or aromatic allure, oregano continues to inspire and enrich culinary traditions and wellness practices.

Plant Profile: Thyme

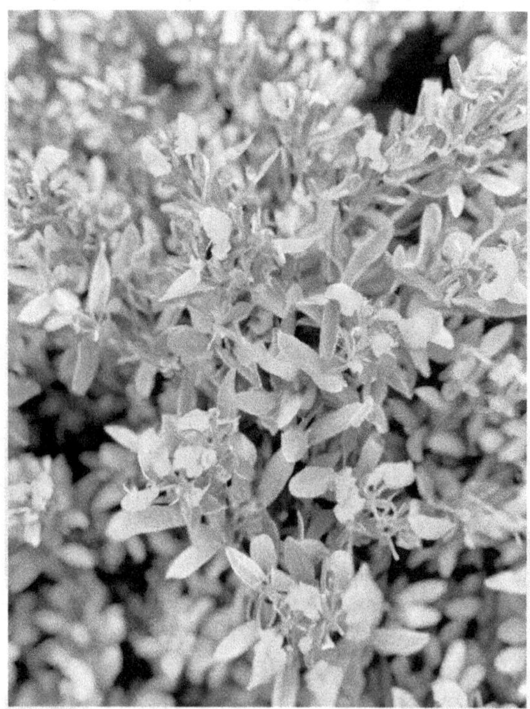

Thyme, renowned for its aromatic foliage and medicinal properties, belongs to the genus Thymus within the Lamiaceae family. In this profile, we explore the identification, parts used, cultivation, properties, and diverse uses of thyme, highlighting its culinary importance and therapeutic benefits.

Identification

- Appearance: Thyme is a perennial herb with small, elliptical leaves that grow in clusters along woody stems. The leaves are usually gray-green to dark green, and some varieties may have variegated foliage. Thyme plants produce tiny, tubular flowers that range in color from white to pink or lavender.

- Fragrance: Thyme leaves release a strong, herbal aroma when crushed, attributed to its essential oils rich in thymol, carvacrol, and linalool.

Parts Used

- Leaves: Thyme leaves are the primary part used for culinary and medicinal purposes. They are harvested throughout the growing season for their intense flavor and aromatic oils. Fresh leaves can be used immediately, while dried leaves retain their potency for long-term storage.

- Essential Oil: Thyme essential oil is extracted from the leaves and flowering tops through steam distillation. It contains potent aromatic compounds that contribute to its therapeutic properties.

Cultivation

Thyme is native to the Mediterranean region but is cultivated worldwide for its culinary appeal and health benefits. Here are key cultivation tips:

- Climate: Thyme thrives in warm, sunny climates with well-draining soil. It prefers temperatures between 60-80°F (15-27°C) and is tolerant of drought once established.

- Soil: Plant thyme in sandy, loamy soil with a pH level between 6.0 and 8.0. Amend the soil with organic matter such as compost to improve fertility and drainage.
- Watering: Allow the soil to dry out slightly between waterings. Water thyme at the base to prevent fungal diseases and promote healthy root development.
- Propagation: Thyme is propagated from seeds, cuttings, or division of established plants. Sow seeds indoors in early spring or directly in the garden after the last frost. Cuttings root easily in water or moist soil.

Properties

- Antimicrobial: Thyme exhibits strong antimicrobial properties due to its high content of thymol and carvacrol. It helps inhibit the growth of bacteria, fungi, and parasites.
- Antioxidant: Thyme is rich in antioxidants such as flavonoids and phenolic compounds, which protect cells from oxidative stress caused by free radicals.
- Anti-inflammatory: The anti-inflammatory compounds in thyme, including rosmarinic acid, help reduce inflammation in the body. It is beneficial for respiratory conditions and arthritis.
- Expectorant: Thyme acts as an expectorant, promoting the clearance of mucus from the lungs and airways. It is used to alleviate coughs and congestion.

Uses

- Culinary Delights: Thyme leaves are used fresh or dried to flavor a variety of savory dishes, including meats, soups, stews, sauces, and roasted vegetables. It adds a subtle, earthy flavor and aroma to culinary creations.
- Herbal Teas: Thyme tea is brewed from fresh or dried leaves and consumed to soothe sore throats, alleviate respiratory infections, and support digestive health. It has a warming and comforting effect.
- Medicinal Remedies: Thyme extracts or tinctures are used in herbal medicine to treat respiratory infections, bronchitis, and digestive disorders. It is also applied topically to relieve minor skin irritations.
- Aromatherapy: Thyme essential oil is diffused or used in massage blends to reduce stress, boost mental clarity, and enhance respiratory function.

Thyme's aromatic leaves and potent health benefits have made it a cherished herb in culinary and medicinal traditions worldwide. Whether enjoyed for its culinary versatility, therapeutic properties, or aromatic allure, thyme continues to inspire and enrich wellness practices.

Plant Profile: Nettle

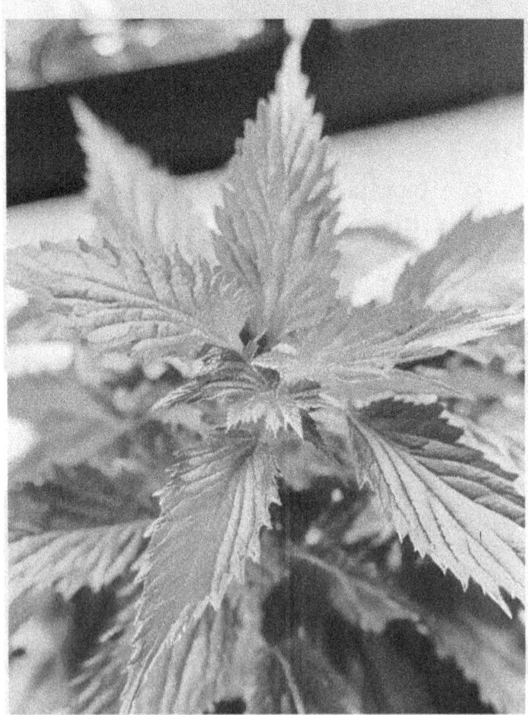

Nettle, known for its stinging hairs and medicinal properties, belongs to the genus Urtica within the Urticaceae family. In this profile, we explore the identification, parts used, cultivation, properties, and diverse uses of nettle, highlighting its nutritional richness and therapeutic benefits.

Identification

- **Appearance:** Nettle is a perennial herbaceous plant with serrated, heart-shaped leaves that grow opposite each other along square stems. The leaves and stems are covered with tiny stinging hairs that release histamine and other chemicals upon contact, causing a stinging sensation on the skin. Nettle flowers are small and greenish-white, arranged in dense clusters.
- **Habitat:** Nettle thrives in nutrient-rich soils and is commonly found in temperate regions worldwide. It grows prolifically in disturbed areas, along riverbanks, and in woodland clearings.

Parts Used

- **Leaves:** Nettle leaves are the primary part used for culinary and medicinal purposes. They are harvested in spring before flowering for optimal tenderness and nutrient content. Fresh leaves can be steamed, sautéed, or brewed into tea, while dried leaves are used for infusions and extracts.
- **Root:** Nettle roots are harvested in late fall or early spring when the plant is dormant. They are dried and used to make extracts or tinctures valued for their therapeutic properties.

> Seeds: Nettle seeds are less commonly used but are harvested from mature plants for their potential health benefits, including as a tonic for overall health.

Cultivation

Nettle is native to Europe, Asia, and North America but is now naturalized in many regions. Here are key cultivation tips:

> Soil: Plant nettle in rich, moist soil with good drainage. It thrives in nitrogen-rich soils and benefits from organic matter such as compost.

> Sunlight: Nettle grows best in partial shade to full sun. It can tolerate various light conditions but may grow more vigorously in partial shade.

> Propagation: Nettle spreads via seeds and rhizomes. Direct sow seeds in early spring or propagate from root divisions in autumn. Ensure plants have enough space to spread, as they can become invasive in favorable conditions.

> Maintenance: Harvest nettle leaves before flowering to avoid bitterness. Wear gloves when handling fresh leaves to avoid stings from the hairs.

Properties

> Nutritional: Nettle leaves are rich in vitamins (A, C, K), minerals (iron, calcium, magnesium), and chlorophyll, making them a valuable dietary supplement.

> Anti-inflammatory: Nettle contains bioactive compounds such as flavonoids and phenolic acids that help reduce inflammation in the body. It is used to alleviate symptoms of arthritis, allergies, and skin conditions.

> Diuretic: Nettle has diuretic properties that support kidney function and help flush toxins from the body. It is used to treat urinary tract infections and edema.

> Antioxidant: The antioxidants in nettle, including carotenoids and vitamin C, protect cells from oxidative stress and promote overall health.

Uses

> Culinary: Nettle leaves are cooked and used as a nutritious vegetable in soups, stews, and teas. They have a mild, spinach-like flavor when cooked and are highly nutritious.

> Herbal Teas: Nettle leaf tea is brewed from fresh or dried leaves and consumed for its nutritive benefits, including as a tonic for overall health and vitality.

> Medicinal Remedies: Nettle extracts or tinctures are used in herbal medicine to treat

allergies, hay fever, arthritis, and anemia. It is also applied topically to soothe skin irritations and promote wound healing.

> **Textiles:** Historically, nettle fibers were used to make durable fabrics, ropes, and paper due to their strength and flexibility.

Nettle's nutritional richness and therapeutic versatility have made it a revered herb throughout history. Whether consumed for its culinary benefits, medicinal properties, or practical uses, nettle continues to be valued for its role in promoting health and well-being.

Plant Profile: Holy Basil (Tulsi)

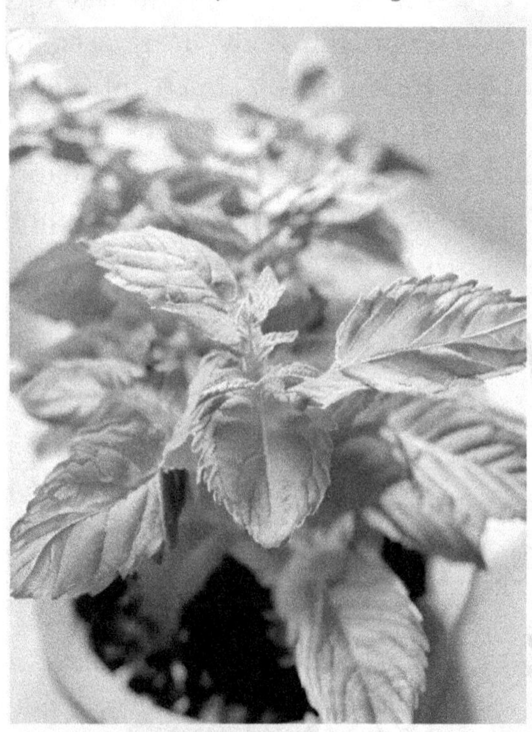

Holy Basil, also known as Tulsi, holds sacred status in Hindu culture and is esteemed for its medicinal properties. Belonging to the Ocimum genus within the Lamiaceae family, Tulsi is revered for its aromatic leaves and therapeutic benefits. In this profile, we delve into the identification, parts used, cultivation, properties, and diverse uses of Holy Basil.

Identification

> **Appearance:** Holy Basil is a perennial herb with fragrant, green or purple-hued leaves that are oval and serrated. The plant grows upright, reaching heights of up to 1-2 feet (30-60 cm). It produces small, purple or white flowers arranged in spikes that attract pollinators.

> **Fragrance:** The leaves of Holy Basil emit a strong, sweet aroma with notes of clove and pepper when crushed, owing to its rich essential oil content.

Parts Used

> **Leaves:** The leaves of Holy Basil are the primary part used for medicinal purposes. They are harvested throughout the growing season for their potent essential oils and

bioactive compounds. Fresh leaves are preferred for immediate use, while dried leaves are stored for longer-term medicinal preparations.

➢ Seeds: Holy Basil seeds are less commonly used but can be harvested and dried for future propagation or medicinal purposes.

Cultivation

Holy Basil is native to Southeast Asia but is cultivated worldwide for its medicinal and cultural significance. Here are key cultivation tips:

➢ Climate: Holy Basil thrives in warm, tropical climates with temperatures between 70-90°F (21-32°C). It requires full sun for optimal growth but can tolerate partial shade.

➢ Soil: Plant Holy Basil in well-draining, fertile soil with a pH between 6.0 and 7.5. Amend the soil with organic matter such as compost to enhance nutrient retention and drainage.

➢ Watering: Keep the soil consistently moist but not waterlogged. Water Holy Basil at the base to prevent fungal diseases and promote healthy root development.

➢ Propagation: Holy Basil is propagated from seeds or cuttings. Sow seeds indoors in early spring or directly in the garden after the last frost. Cuttings root easily in water or moist soil.

Properties

➢ Adaptogen: Holy Basil is classified as an adaptogen, helping the body cope with stress and promoting balance. It supports adrenal function and helps mitigate the effects of stress on the body.

➢ Antioxidant: The leaves of Holy Basil are rich in antioxidants such as flavonoids and phenolic compounds, which protect cells from oxidative damage caused by free radicals.

➢ Anti-inflammatory: Holy Basil contains eugenol, rosmarinic acid, and other anti-inflammatory compounds that help reduce inflammation and support joint health.

➢ Antimicrobial: Holy Basil exhibits antimicrobial properties, inhibiting the growth of bacteria, fungi, and other pathogens. It is used to treat infections and promote wound healing.

Uses

➢ Culinary: Holy Basil leaves are used fresh or dried to add flavor to Thai and Indian cuisines, including curries, stir-fries, soups, and salads. It adds a unique, peppery-sweet flavor to dishes.

- ➢ **Herbal Teas:** Tulsi tea is brewed from fresh or dried Holy Basil leaves and consumed for its calming effects, respiratory support, and digestive benefits. It has a refreshing and uplifting taste.
- ➢ **Medicinal Remedies:** Holy Basil extracts, tinctures, or teas are used in Ayurvedic and herbal medicine to alleviate stress, promote mental clarity, support cardiovascular health, and boost immunity.
- ➢ **Religious and Cultural Significance:** Holy Basil is revered in Hindu culture and is often grown near temples and homes. It is used in religious rituals, prayers, and ceremonies to invoke spiritual blessings and purification.

Holy Basil, or Tulsi, embodies the rich tradition of Ayurvedic medicine and cultural reverence in Southeast Asia. Whether cherished for its culinary uses, medicinal benefits, or spiritual significance, Holy Basil continues to inspire and nurture both body and spirit.

Plant Profile: Milk Thistle

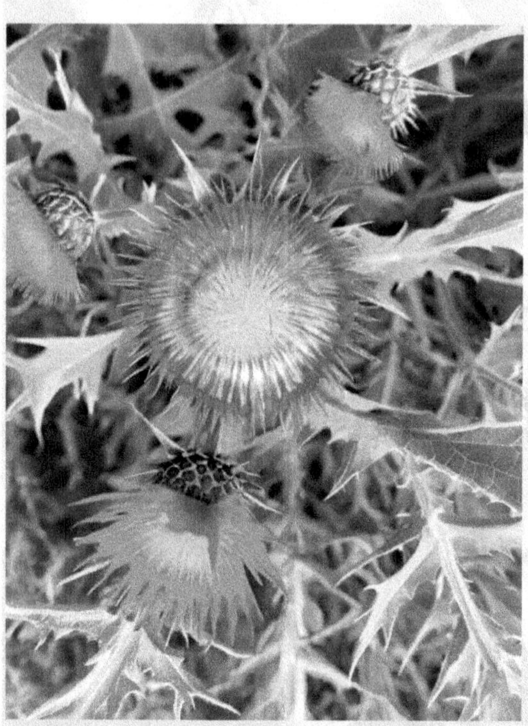

Milk Thistle, scientifically known as Silybum marianum, is a flowering herbaceous plant belonging to the Asteraceae family. Renowned for its distinctive appearance and medicinal properties, Milk Thistle has been used for centuries in traditional medicine. In this profile, we explore the identification, parts used, cultivation, properties, and diverse uses of Milk Thistle.

Identification

- ➢ **Appearance:** Milk Thistle is characterized by its tall, spiny stems that can reach heights of up to 6 feet (1.8 meters). The plant features large, glossy, dark green leaves with white veins that have a milky-white marbling effect, hence its name. The stems and leaves are adorned with sharp spines. Milk Thistle blooms with striking purple to pinkish flowers that resemble thistle heads, each flowerhead containing numerous spiky bracts.

- ➤ **Habitat:** Native to the Mediterranean region, Milk Thistle now grows in temperate regions worldwide. It thrives in dry, rocky soils and is often found in disturbed habitats, along roadsides, and in fields.

Parts Used

- ➤ **Seeds:** The seeds of Milk Thistle are the most commonly used part for medicinal purposes. They are harvested when fully ripe and dried for extraction. The seeds contain a bioactive complex known as silymarin, which is the primary therapeutic component.
- ➤ **Leaves:** While less commonly used than the seeds, Milk Thistle leaves can be harvested for medicinal preparations. They are typically dried and used as a tea or in herbal formulations.

Cultivation

Milk Thistle is cultivated for both its ornamental value and medicinal benefits. Here are key cultivation tips:

- ➤ **Climate:** Milk Thistle thrives in full sun to partial shade. It prefers dry, well-drained soils and can tolerate poor soil conditions.
- ➤ **Propagation:** Milk Thistle is propagated from seeds, which should be sown directly into the garden in early spring after the last frost. The seeds germinate best in cooler temperatures.
- ➤ **Watering:** Once established, Milk Thistle is drought-tolerant and requires minimal watering. Avoid overwatering, as it can lead to root rot.
- ➤ **Maintenance:** Remove spent flower heads to prevent self-seeding and maintain the plant's appearance. Wear gloves when handling Milk Thistle due to its spiny nature.

Properties

- ➤ **Hepatoprotective:** Milk Thistle is best known for its hepatoprotective properties, primarily attributed to silymarin. It supports liver health by promoting regeneration of liver cells, protecting against toxins, and enhancing detoxification processes.
- ➤ **Antioxidant:** Silymarin and other flavonoids in Milk Thistle exhibit strong antioxidant activity, scavenging free radicals and reducing oxidative stress in the body.
- ➤ **Anti-inflammatory:** Milk Thistle has anti-inflammatory properties that may help

reduce inflammation in conditions such as arthritis and digestive disorders.
- ➤ **Choleretic:** Milk Thistle stimulates bile production and flow, aiding in digestion and promoting gallbladder health.

Uses

- ➤ **Liver Support:** Milk Thistle is widely used to support liver function and treat liver conditions such as hepatitis, cirrhosis, and fatty liver disease. It helps protect the liver from damage and supports its natural detoxification processes.
- ➤ **Digestive Health:** The choleretic properties of Milk Thistle promote healthy digestion and alleviate symptoms of indigestion, bloating, and constipation.
- ➤ **Antioxidant Support:** Regular use of Milk Thistle may help protect against oxidative damage and support overall antioxidant defenses in the body.
- ➤ **Skin Health:** Milk Thistle extracts or topical preparations are used to treat skin conditions such as acne, eczema, and psoriasis due to its anti-inflammatory and antioxidant properties.

Milk Thistle's robust medicinal properties and striking appearance make it a valuable herb in both traditional and modern herbal medicine. Whether used to support liver health, enhance digestion, or promote overall well-being, Milk Thistle continues to be cherished for its therapeutic benefits.

3

Cultivating and Harvesting Herbs

Cultivating and harvesting herbs is an enriching and rewarding practice that blends the art of gardening with the science of herbal medicine. This chapter delves into the essential principles of growing and harvesting herbs, whether you have a sprawling garden or a cozy indoor space. By understanding the fundamental techniques and requirements, you'll be able to nurture a variety of herbs that can enhance your health, cuisine, and overall well-being.

Growing herbs starts with grasping the basics: the types of soil, sunlight, and water each herb requires. Different herbs have unique needs, and tailoring your approach to meet these requirements can make all the difference in achieving a thriving herb garden. Whether you're growing common kitchen herbs like basil and rosemary or medicinal plants like echinacea and valerian, knowing how to create the ideal conditions for each plant is crucial.

Creating an herbal garden can be a versatile endeavor, accommodating both indoor and outdoor settings. For those with ample outdoor space, a dedicated herb garden can become a sanctuary of aromas and colors, attracting beneficial insects and providing a constant supply of fresh herbs. For indoor gardeners, container gardening offers a practical solution, allowing you to grow herbs on windowsills, balconies, or small patios. We'll explore tips and techniques for both scenarios, ensuring that your herbs receive the care and attention they need, regardless of where they're planted.

Harvesting herbs at the right time is an art that maximizes their potency and flavor. Understanding the optimal harvest times for various herbs, as well as the best techniques for cutting and preserving them, ensures that you make the most of your efforts. We'll cover methods for drying, freezing, and storing herbs, so you can enjoy their benefits long after they've been harvested.

Sustainable and ethical wildcrafting practices are also an essential aspect of herbalism. Wildcrafting involves harvesting herbs from their natural habitats, and doing so responsibly is crucial for maintaining ecological balance. This chapter will provide guidelines on how to wildcraft herbs sustainably, ensuring that natural populations remain healthy and abundant for future generations.

By mastering the skills of cultivating and harvesting herbs, you'll be able to create a personal apothecary, filled with the therapeutic and culinary treasures of nature. This chapter will equip you with the knowledge and confidence to grow and harvest herbs successfully, bringing the wisdom of herbalism into your home and daily life.

Basic Principles of Growing Herbs

1. Growing herbs is not merely about planting seeds; it's a harmonious dance between soil, sunlight, water, and mindful nurturing. Understanding the basic principles sets the foundation for successful herb cultivation:
2. Soil Health: Herbs thrive in well-draining, nutrient-rich soil. Learn how to amend your soil with compost and organic matter to provide the ideal growing environment.
3. Sunlight Requirements: Most herbs prefer full sun, while some thrive in partial shade. Discover how to position your garden to maximize sunlight exposure based on herb varieties.
4. Watering Techniques: Strike the delicate balance between hydration and drainage. Explore watering schedules and techniques to ensure herbs receive adequate moisture without waterlogging.
5. Seasonal Considerations: Tailor your cultivation practices to each season. From sowing seeds in spring to protecting tender herbs from frost in winter, align your gardening efforts with nature's rhythm.

Creating an Herbal Garden: Indoor and Outdoor Tips

Whether you have a spacious backyard or a cozy windowsill, creating an herbal garden opens a gateway to sustainable living and holistic wellness:

Indoor Herb Gardens: Transform your kitchen or living space into a thriving herb sanctuary. Learn how to select containers, choose suitable herbs for indoor growth, and provide optimal lighting and humidity levels.

Outdoor Herb Gardens: Harness the power of outdoor spaces to cultivate a diverse array of herbs. Discover companion planting techniques, raised bed gardening tips, and ways to attract beneficial insects.

Vertical Gardening: Maximize limited space with vertical gardening solutions. Explore creative herb trellising, hanging baskets, and tower gardens to cultivate herbs in urban settings or small yards.

Harvesting Techniques: Delve into the art of harvesting herbs at peak potency. From pruning methods to timing harvests for maximum flavor and medicinal benefits, master the delicate balance between growth and sustainability.

Harvesting and Storing Herbs

Harvesting herbs is a culmination of patience, observation, and a deep connection to the earth's rhythms. As we explore the art of gathering herbs at their peak and preserving their vitality, we embark on a journey that honors sustainability, herbal wisdom, and the art of preservation.

Harvesting Herbs: Timing and Techniques

The key to harvesting herbs lies in timing—the moment when their essential oils and medicinal properties are at their peak. Whether you're harvesting from your garden or foraging in the wild, mastering these techniques ensures optimal flavor and efficacy:

1. Timing: Harvest herbs in the morning after dew has dried but before the sun's heat diminishes their essential oils. For culinary herbs, gather them just before they flower for the best flavor. Medicinal herbs often require harvesting at specific stages of growth, such as before flowering or when seeds are ripe.
2. Tools: Use sharp, clean scissors or pruning shears to cut herbs, ensuring a clean cut that promotes healthy regrowth. For delicate herbs, gently pluck leaves by hand to avoid damaging the plant.
3. Cutting Techniques: When harvesting leafy herbs such as basil or mint, cut stems just above a pair of leaves to encourage bushy growth. For woody herbs like rosemary or thyme, trim just above a node to stimulate new growth from the base.

Storing Herbs: Preserving Freshness and Potency

Once harvested, proper storage is essential to maintain herbs' freshness, flavor, and medicinal properties over time. Follow these guidelines to preserve herbs for culinary delights and herbal remedies:

1. Fresh Herbs: Immediately after harvest, rinse herbs gently with cold water to remove dirt and debris. Shake off excess moisture and allow them to air dry on a clean towel. Store fresh herbs in the refrigerator, either loosely wrapped in a damp paper towel inside a plastic bag or upright in a glass of water like fresh flowers.
2. Drying Herbs: Air drying is a traditional method for preserving herbs' potency. Tie small bunches of herbs with twine and hang them upside down in a warm, dry place with good airflow. Once completely dry, store herbs in

airtight containers away from direct sunlight to maintain flavor and aroma.

3. Freezing Herbs: Preserve herbs by freezing them in ice cube trays filled with water or olive oil. Alternatively, finely chop herbs and freeze them in sealed plastic bags or containers. Frozen herbs retain their flavor well and are convenient for cooking throughout the year.

4. Herbal Infusions: Create herbal vinegars, oils, or tinctures to extend the shelf life of fresh herbs while extracting their medicinal properties. Fill clean glass jars with herbs and cover completely with vinegar, oil, or alcohol. Seal tightly and store in a cool, dark place for several weeks before straining.

Sustainable and Ethical Wildcrafting Practices

Wildcrafting, the practice of harvesting plants from their natural habitats, requires careful consideration of sustainability and ethical principles. When foraging for wild herbs, adopt these practices to ensure the health of ecosystems and respect for plant communities:

1. Identification: Thoroughly research and correctly identify wild plants before harvesting. Use reliable field guides or consult with experienced herbalists to avoid harvesting endangered or protected species.

2. Harvesting Mindfully: Harvest only what you need and leave ample plants to regenerate and support local wildlife. Practice selective harvesting to minimize impact on wild populations, focusing on abundant species and avoiding disturbance to sensitive habitats.

3. Respect for Ecosystems: Harvest with reverence for the natural environment. Avoid damaging plants, disrupting soil, or disturbing wildlife habitats. Leave no trace of your presence and tread lightly to preserve biodiversity and ecological balance.

4. Cultural Sensitivity: Respect indigenous traditions and cultural practices related to wildcrafting. Seek permission when foraging on private land and honor local regulations regarding plant harvesting and conservation.

Harvesting and storing herbs is not just a practical skill but a profound journey into the heart of herbalism and sustainability. As we cultivate a deeper connection to nature's bounty, we honor ancient traditions and nurture our well-being with each herb harvested mindfully.

Let us continue to tread lightly on the Earth, fostering a harmonious relationship with plants and ecosystems. Through mindful harvesting, thoughtful stewardship, and the preservation of herbal wisdom, we ensure that future generations can also enjoy the gifts of nature's healing bounty.

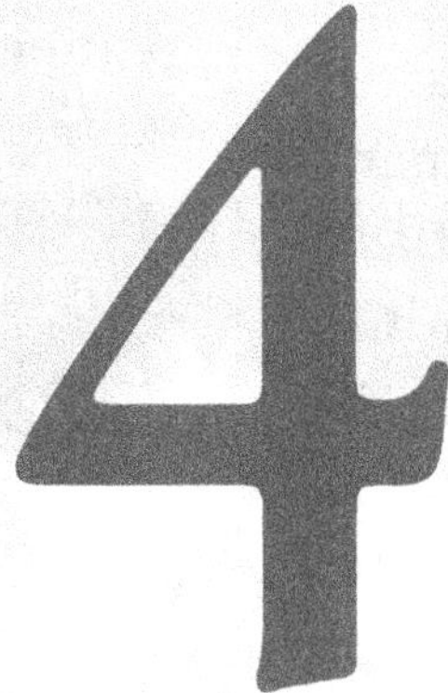

4

Safety and Precautions

Herbal remedies offer a natural and effective way to support health and wellness, drawing on centuries of traditional knowledge and modern research. However, just as with any form of medicine, it is crucial to approach herbalism with a clear understanding of safety and precautions. This chapter is dedicated to providing essential guidelines to ensure the responsible and informed use of herbal treatments.

Understanding herbal contraindications is fundamental for anyone interested in using plant-based remedies. Certain herbs may interact with medications or specific health conditions, making it important to be aware of potential risks. Recognizing these contraindications helps prevent adverse reactions and ensures that herbs are used in a manner that supports overall health.

Managing side effects is another critical aspect of herbal safety. While many herbs are gentle and have few side effects, others can cause reactions, especially when used inappropriately or in excessive amounts. Learning to identify and manage these side effects allows for the safe and effective use of herbal remedies.

The topic of herb-drug interactions cannot be overstated. Many herbs can interact with pharmaceutical drugs, either enhancing or diminishing their effects. This chapter provides comprehensive information on the most common interactions, helping readers make informed decisions and consult healthcare professionals when necessary.

Safe dosage guidelines are also essential for the effective use of herbs. Unlike standardized pharmaceuticals, the potency of herbs can vary widely. This chapter offers practical advice on determining appropriate dosages, ensuring that the benefits of herbs are maximized while minimizing the risk of adverse effects.

By understanding these key aspects of herbal safety, readers can confidently incorporate herbs into their wellness routines. This chapter serves as a vital resource, providing the knowledge needed to use herbal remedies responsibly and effectively, ultimately enhancing health and well-being through informed choices.

Understanding Herbal Contraindications

Herbal medicine, with its rich tradition and holistic approach, offers a myriad of benefits for health and well-being. However, just as herbs can support and heal, they can also interact with medications, conditions, or individual constitutions in ways that require careful consideration:

1. Individual Variability: Every person is unique, with varying health histories, sensitivities, and medications. Understanding herbal contraindications involves recognizing which herbs may not be suitable for certain individuals due to pre-existing health conditions, allergies, or ongoing treatments.
2. Interaction with Medications: Some herbs may interact with prescription or over-the-counter medications, altering their effectiveness or causing adverse effects. It's essential to consult with healthcare providers to understand potential interactions and adjust herbal treatments accordingly.
3. Specific Health Conditions: Certain herbs may exacerbate conditions such as hypertension, liver disorders, or hormonal imbalances. Knowledge of contraindications helps herbalists tailor treatments to promote safe and effective outcomes while respecting individual health needs.

Recognizing and Managing Side Effects

While herbal remedies are generally considered safe when used appropriately, they can occasionally produce side effects, particularly with improper dosage or prolonged use. Recognizing and managing these effects is crucial for maintaining wellness and promoting responsible herbal practice:

1. Common Side Effects: Learn to identify common side effects such as digestive disturbances, allergic reactions, or mild headaches. Prompt recognition allows for timely adjustments in dosage or formulation to minimize discomfort and ensure continued safety.
2. Monitoring and Feedback: Encourage clients or individuals using herbal remedies to provide feedback on their experiences. This ongoing dialogue enables herbalists to monitor reactions, adjust treatment plans, and address concerns promptly.
3. Professional Guidance: Seek guidance from qualified herbalists or healthcare providers when managing side effects, especially if symptoms persist or worsen.

Collaboration ensures holistic care and enhances safety in herbal practice.

In the realm of herbalism, safety is not merely a precaution but a foundational principle that underpins effective and ethical practice. By integrating knowledge of herbal contraindications and vigilant monitoring of side effects, herbalists uphold standards of care that prioritize client well-being and promote sustainable health outcomes.

As you navigate the intricate landscape of herbal remedies, may this chapter empower you to practice with confidence and compassion. By embracing safety measures and honoring individual health considerations, we nurture a culture of informed herbal practice that respects the potency and potential of nature's healing gifts.

Herb-Drug Interactions

Herbal medicine offers a tapestry of natural remedies that complement conventional healthcare practices. However, understanding herb-drug interactions is crucial to ensure safe and effective integration of herbal therapies with pharmaceutical treatments. This section explores the complexities of herb-drug interactions and empowers practitioners with essential knowledge for informed practice.

Understanding Herb-Drug Interactions

Herb-drug interactions occur when substances in herbs affect the pharmacokinetics (absorption, distribution, metabolism, and excretion) or pharmacodynamics (effects) of medications. These interactions can potentiate or inhibit drug actions, alter drug levels in the body, or lead to unexpected side effects:

1. Mechanisms of Interaction: Herbs may interact with medications by affecting enzymes in the liver (which metabolize drugs), altering absorption in the gut, or influencing drug transport mechanisms. Examples include St. John's wort, which accelerates the metabolism of certain medications, and grapefruit juice, which inhibits enzyme activity, affecting drug absorption.

2. Common Interactions: Identify common herb-drug interactions to mitigate risks. For instance, ginkgo biloba may increase bleeding risk when used with blood-thinning medications like warfarin, while garlic

supplements may interact with anticoagulants, affecting blood clotting times.

3. Individualized Assessment: Conduct thorough assessments of patients' medication histories, including herbal supplements, to identify potential interactions. Collaborate with healthcare providers to adjust treatment plans and monitor patient responses to minimize risks and optimize therapeutic outcomes.

Safe Dosage Guidelines: Balancing Efficacy and Safety

Safe dosage guidelines are fundamental in herbal practice to ensure therapeutic efficacy while preventing adverse effects. Herbalists rely on evidence-based dosing principles and individualized assessments to tailor treatments to each person's unique health profile:

1. Dosage Considerations: Consider factors such as age, weight, health status, and sensitivity when determining herbal dosages. Start with low doses and gradually titrate upward to gauge individual responses and tolerance levels.

2. Herbal Formulations: Choose appropriate formulations (e.g., teas, tinctures, capsules) based on the herb's bioavailability and desired therapeutic effect. Adjust dosages accordingly for acute conditions, chronic management, or supportive care.

3. Monitoring and Adjustment: Monitor patient responses closely and adjust dosages as needed to achieve therapeutic goals. Educate patients on self-monitoring for adverse effects and encourage open communication to optimize treatment outcomes.

In herbalism, knowledge of herb-drug interactions and adherence to safe dosage guidelines form the cornerstone of responsible practice. By integrating these principles into clinical decision-making, herbalists uphold standards of care that prioritize patient safety, collaboration with healthcare providers, and holistic well-being.

As stewards of herbal wisdom and agents of health promotion, may this chapter empower you to navigate the complexities of herb-drug interactions with confidence and compassion. By embracing informed practice, we forge pathways to integrated healthcare that honor the synergistic potential of natural and pharmaceutical therapies.

5

Herbal Recipes for Common Ailments

Welcome to the chapter dedicated to herbal recipes for common ailments—a treasury of natural solutions crafted to alleviate everyday health challenges. In this section, we explore the art of blending medicinal herbs into delicious and effective remedies tailored to support holistic wellness.

What is Herbal Recipes for Common Ailments?

Herbal recipes for common ailments encompass a diverse array of preparations designed to address a spectrum of health concerns naturally. From soothing teas and healing salves to potent tinctures and comforting soups, these recipes draw on centuries of herbal wisdom to promote well-being and vitality.

Throughout this chapter, you'll discover practical and accessible recipes curated to empower you on your journey toward optimal health. Each recipe combines specific herbs renowned for their therapeutic properties, offering gentle yet effective relief for ailments ranging from digestive discomfort and stress to respiratory issues and skin conditions.

Join me as we unlock the transformative potential of herbs, blending tradition with innovation to cultivate resilience and vitality. Whether you're seeking immune support, digestive ease, or emotional balance, these herbal recipes invite you to harness the healing power of nature in your daily wellness rituals.

Recipes for Digestive Health

Digestive health is foundational to overall well-being, influencing everything from nutrient absorption to immune function and mood regulation. The recipes curated here are crafted with care, combining traditional herbal knowledge with modern culinary sensibilities to create dishes that not only taste delightful but also support optimal digestive function.

Whether you're seeking relief from occasional discomfort, aiming to enhance digestive efficiency, or simply nurturing gut health as part of your wellness routine, these recipes offer practical and delicious solutions. From soothing herbal teas and digestion-enhancing soups to probiotic-rich salads and gut-supporting tonics, each recipe invites you to harness the power of herbs and wholesome ingredients to cultivate a happy, balanced digestive system.

Peppermint Tummy Tea Recipe

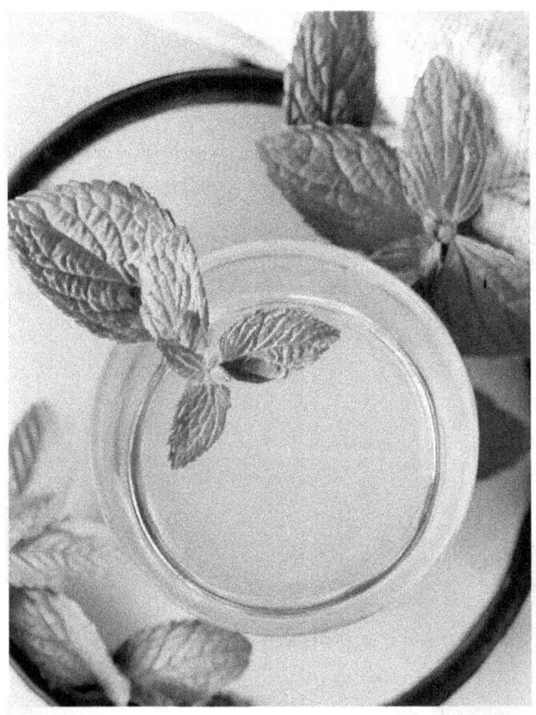

Time of Preparation: 10 minutes

Serving Unit: 1 cup

Ingredients:

- 1 tablespoon dried peppermint leaves (or 3 tablespoons fresh peppermint leaves)
- 1 cup water
- Optional: honey or lemon to taste

Procedures:

1. Boil Water: Bring 1 cup of water to a boil in a small saucepan or kettle.
2. Prepare Peppermint: If using fresh peppermint leaves, crush them gently to release their oils. If using dried leaves, place them in a teapot or heat-resistant container.
3. Steep: Pour the boiling water over the peppermint leaves.
4. Timing: Cover and steep for 5-10 minutes, depending on desired strength.
5. Strain and Serve: Strain the tea into a cup to remove the peppermint leaves. Add honey or lemon if desired for sweetness and flavor.

Tips and Tricks:

- For a stronger tea, steep the peppermint leaves for a longer duration.
- Use organic peppermint leaves if possible to avoid pesticides and chemicals.
- Adjust sweetness with honey or acidity with lemon according to personal taste preferences.

Nutritional Value (per serving):

- Calories: 0
- Carbohydrates: 0g
- Fat: 0g
- Protein: 0g
- Vitamin C: 0mcg

Health Benefits:

- Digestive Aid: Peppermint is known for its ability to soothe digestive issues such as indigestion, bloating, and gas.
- Antispasmodic Properties: Helps to relax the muscles of the digestive tract, easing cramps and discomfort.

- ➢ Anti-inflammatory: Reduces inflammation in the gastrointestinal tract, supporting overall digestive health.

Storage and Heating Requirements:

- ➢ Storage: Store any leftover tea in a sealed container in the refrigerator for up to 24 hours.
- ➢ Heating: Reheat gently on the stovetop or in the microwave until warm, but not boiling, to preserve its beneficial properties.

Enjoy your Peppermint Tummy Tea as a soothing and refreshing remedy for digestive wellness. Embrace its natural goodness and therapeutic benefits as part of your daily health routine.

Ginger Digestive Syrup Recipe

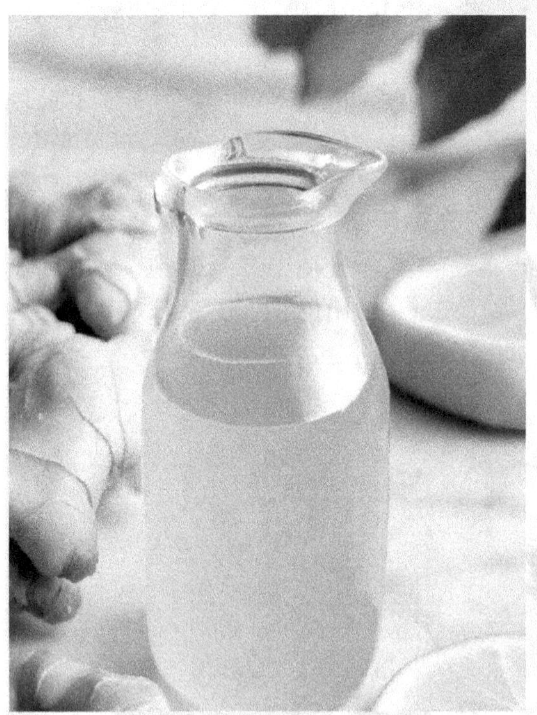

Time of Preparation: 20 minutes

Serving Unit: 1 tablespoon

Ingredients:

- ➢ 1 cup water
- ➢ 1/2 cup fresh ginger root, peeled and grated
- ➢ 1/2 cup honey
- ➢ Optional: lemon juice to taste

Procedures:

1. Prepare Ginger: Peel and grate the fresh ginger root to yield approximately 1/2 cup.
2. Boil Water: In a small saucepan, bring 1 cup of water to a boil.
3. Infuse Ginger: Add the grated ginger to the boiling water. Reduce heat and simmer for 10-15 minutes, allowing the ginger to infuse into the water.
4. Strain: Remove the saucepan from heat and let the ginger steep for an additional 5 minutes. Strain the ginger pieces from the liquid using a fine mesh sieve or cheesecloth, pressing gently to extract all liquid.
5. Add Honey: While the ginger infusion is still warm (not boiling), stir in 1/2 cup of

honey until fully dissolved. Add lemon juice if desired for additional flavor and vitamin C content.

6. Cool and Store: Allow the syrup to cool to room temperature. Transfer to a clean, airtight glass jar or bottle for storage.

Tips and Tricks:

- Adjust the sweetness by varying the amount of honey used according to taste preferences.
- Use raw, unfiltered honey for added nutritional benefits and natural sweetness.
- Store the ginger syrup in the refrigerator to maintain freshness and potency. Use within 1-2 weeks.

Nutritional Value (per serving - 1 tablespoon):

- Calories: 40
- Carbohydrates: 10g
- Sugar: 9g
- Vitamin C: 1mg

Health Benefits:

- Digestive Aid: Ginger promotes digestion by stimulating saliva flow, bile production, and gastric motility, reducing symptoms of indigestion and nausea.
- Anti-inflammatory: Contains gingerol, which exhibits anti-inflammatory properties beneficial for gastrointestinal health.
- Immune Support: Honey and lemon contribute antioxidants and vitamin C, supporting overall immune function and vitality.

Storage and Heating Requirements:

- Storage: Keep the ginger syrup refrigerated in a sealed container. Shake well before use if it separates.
- Heating: Warm gently in a saucepan or microwave before use if desired, but do not boil to preserve the beneficial properties of ginger and honey.

Enjoy your Ginger Digestive Syrup as a natural and effective remedy for digestive comfort and overall wellness. Incorporate it into your daily routine to support healthy digestion and enjoy its soothing benefits.

Fennel Seed Chew Recipe

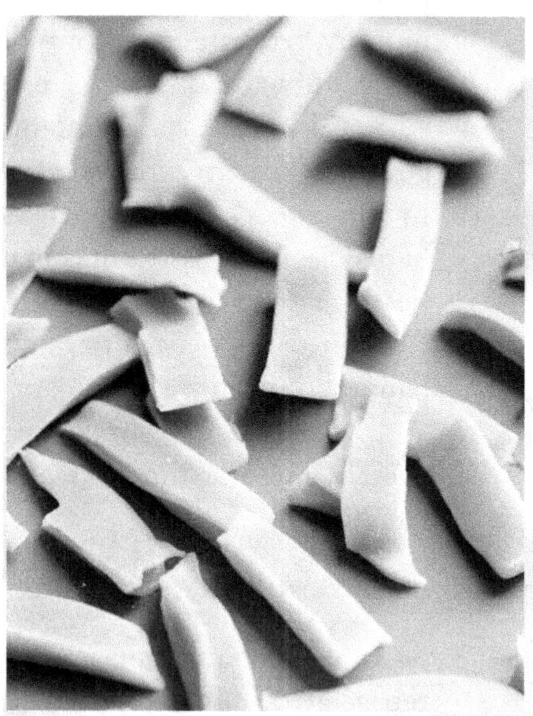

Time of Preparation: 5 minutes

Serving Unit: 1 tablespoon

Ingredients:

- 1 tablespoon whole fennel seeds
- Optional: honey or maple syrup for sweetness

Procedures:

1. Prepare Fennel Seeds: Measure out 1 tablespoon of whole fennel seeds.
2. Optional Toasting (if desired): Heat a dry skillet over medium heat. Add the fennel seeds and toast for 1-2 minutes, stirring frequently, until fragrant. Remove from heat and let cool.
3. Combine Ingredients: Place the fennel seeds in a small bowl. If desired, drizzle with a small amount of honey or maple syrup for added sweetness and flavor.
4. Mix Well: Stir the fennel seeds to coat evenly with the honey or maple syrup, if using.
5. Store and Serve: Transfer the fennel seed chew to a small container with a lid for storage.

Tips and Tricks:

- Customize the sweetness level by adjusting the amount of honey or maple syrup added.
- Toasting the fennel seeds enhances their flavor and aroma but is optional based on personal preference.
- Experiment with different flavors by adding a pinch of sea salt or a sprinkle of cinnamon to the mixture.

Nutritional Value (per serving - 1 tablespoon):

- Calories: 20
- Carbohydrates: 4g
- Fiber: 2g
- Sugar: 0g
- Calcium: 50mcg

Health Benefits:

- Digestive Aid: Fennel seeds contain compounds that help

relax the digestive tract muscles, easing bloating, gas, and indigestion.

➤ **Antioxidant Properties**: Rich in antioxidants, fennel seeds help neutralize harmful free radicals in the body, supporting overall health.

➤ **Oral Health:** Chewing fennel seeds stimulates saliva production, which aids in digestion and promotes oral health.

Storage and Heating Requirements:

➤ **Storage:** Keep the fennel seed chew in a sealed container at room temperature or in the refrigerator for up to 2 weeks.

➤ **Heating:** Serve at room temperature. Avoid heating as it may affect the texture and flavor of the chew.

Enjoy your Fennel Seed Chew as a natural and flavorful way to support digestive health and enjoy its delightful crunch and subtle sweetness. Incorporate it into your daily routine or enjoy it as a post-meal digestive aid.

Recipes for Respiratory Health

Welcome to the world of Recipes for Respiratory Health, where we explore the comforting embrace of nature's remedies for breathing well. In this journey, we delve into the soothing powers of herbs and ingredients crafted into delicious concoctions designed to support your respiratory system. From warming teas that clear the airways to soothing syrups that calm coughs, these recipes are here to nurture and strengthen your respiratory health with every sip and spoonful. Let's embark together on this path to clearer breathing and robust well-being, guided by the wisdom of herbal remedies and the warmth of natural healing.

Eucalyptus Chest Rub

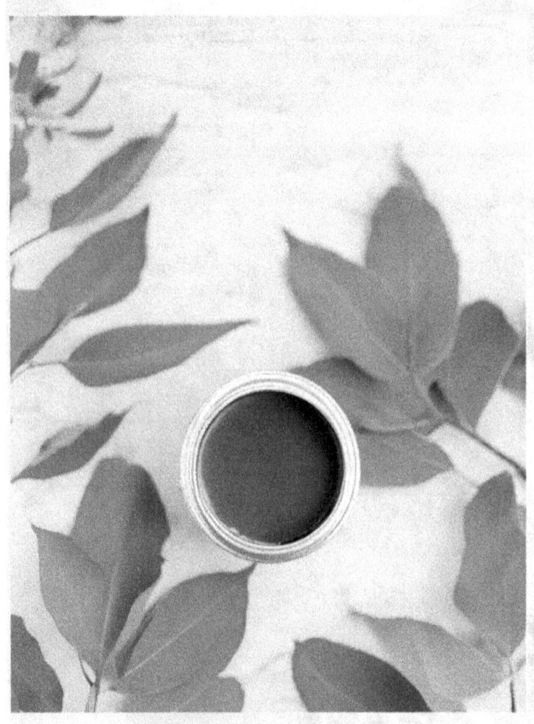

Time of Preparation: 15 minutes

Serving Unit: Varies

Ingredients:

- 1/2 cup coconut oil
- 1/4 cup grated beeswax
- 20 drops eucalyptus essential oil
- 10 drops peppermint essential oil
- 10 drops lavender essential oil

Procedures:

1. Prepare Double Boiler: Fill a saucepan with a couple of inches of water and bring to a simmer. Place a heat-safe bowl on top, ensuring it fits snugly without touching the water.
2. Melt Ingredients: In the bowl, combine coconut oil and grated beeswax. Stir occasionally until fully melted and well combined.
3. Add Essential Oils: Remove the bowl from heat. Quickly stir in eucalyptus, peppermint, and lavender essential oils until evenly distributed.
4. Cool and Pour: Carefully pour the mixture into clean, sterilized jars or tins. Allow it to cool completely at room temperature until solidified.

5. Storage: Seal the jars or tins tightly with lids. Store in a cool, dry place away from direct sunlight.

Tips and Tricks:

- Use organic, unrefined coconut oil for its moisturizing and antibacterial properties.
- Adjust the essential oil amounts to suit personal preferences, ensuring the total drops do not exceed 40 drops per 1/2 cup of carrier oils to maintain safe dilution.
- Test a small amount on the skin to check for sensitivity before extensive use, especially for individuals with sensitive skin or allergies.

Nutritional Value:

- Calories: 0 (for external use)
- Fat: 0g
- Protein: 0g

Health Benefits:

- Respiratory Support: Eucalyptus and peppermint oils are known for their ability to open airways, ease congestion, and relieve cough symptoms.
- Anti-inflammatory: Lavender oil contributes soothing properties, reducing inflammation and promoting relaxation.
- Antimicrobial: Coconut oil and beeswax provide a protective barrier while moisturizing the skin, aiding in skin health.

Storage and Heating Requirements:

- Storage: Keep the eucalyptus chest rub tightly sealed in a cool, dark place. Use within 6 months for optimal freshness and effectiveness.
- Heating: To use, scoop a small amount and warm between palms before gently massaging onto chest and upper back. Avoid direct heat or microwave to prevent altering the consistency and properties of the rub.

Enjoy your Eucalyptus Chest Rub as a comforting and effective remedy for respiratory congestion and support. Embrace its natural healing properties and soothing aroma to promote respiratory health and well-being.

Thyme Cough Syrup

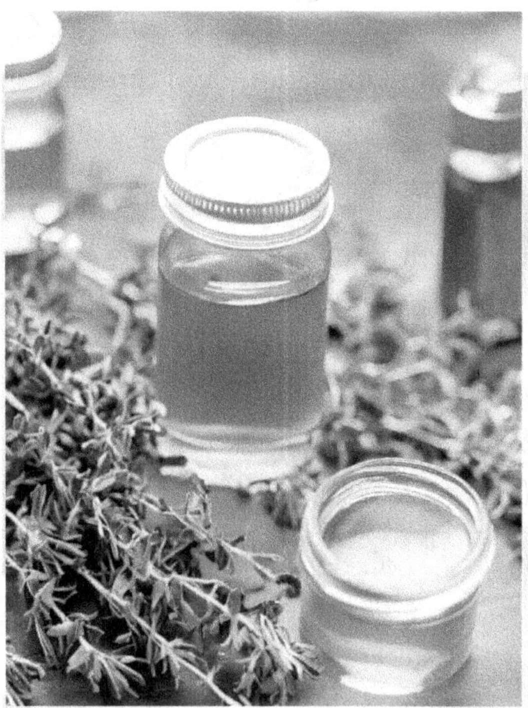

Time of Preparation: 30 minutes

Serving Unit: 1 teaspoon

Ingredients:

- 1 cup water
- 1/4 cup fresh thyme leaves (or 2 tablespoons dried thyme)
- 1/2 cup honey
- Optional: 1-2 tablespoons lemon juice

Procedures:

1. Boil Water: In a small saucepan, bring 1 cup of water to a boil.
2. Add Thyme: Add the fresh thyme leaves (or dried thyme) to the boiling water.
3. Simmer: Reduce heat and let the mixture simmer for 20-25 minutes, allowing the thyme to infuse into the water.
4. Strain: Remove the saucepan from heat and let it cool slightly. Strain the thyme leaves from the liquid using a fine mesh sieve or cheesecloth, pressing gently to extract all liquid.
5. Add Honey: While the thyme infusion is still warm (not boiling), stir in 1/2 cup of honey until fully dissolved. Add lemon juice if desired for additional flavor and vitamin C content.
6. Cool and Store: Allow the syrup to cool to room temperature. Transfer to a clean, airtight glass jar or bottle for storage.

Tips and Tricks:

- Use fresh thyme for a more potent flavor and aroma, but dried thyme works well too.
- Adjust sweetness with more or less honey according to taste preferences.
- Stir in lemon juice at the end for a citrusy twist and added vitamin C, which supports immune health.

Nutritional Value (per serving - 1 teaspoon):

- Calories: 20
- Carbohydrates: 5g
- Sugar: 5g

Health Benefits:

- Cough Relief: Thyme contains compounds like thymol that act as natural cough suppressants and help loosen mucus.
- Antioxidant Properties: Honey and thyme both possess antioxidant properties that support overall immune function and respiratory health.
- Soothing: The warm syrup provides soothing relief to a sore throat and irritated airways.

Storage and Heating Requirements:

- Storage: Keep the thyme cough syrup refrigerated in a sealed container. Use within 1-2 weeks for optimal freshness and effectiveness.
- Heating: Serve at room temperature or warm slightly before use, but do not boil to preserve the beneficial properties of thyme and honey.

Enjoy your Thyme Cough Syrup as a natural and effective remedy for coughs and respiratory discomfort. Incorporate it into your daily routine or use as needed to support respiratory health with the soothing power of thyme and honey.

This recipe combines the therapeutic properties of thyme and honey into a soothing syrup, perfect for alleviating coughs and supporting respiratory wellness naturally.

Licorice Root Throat Lozenges

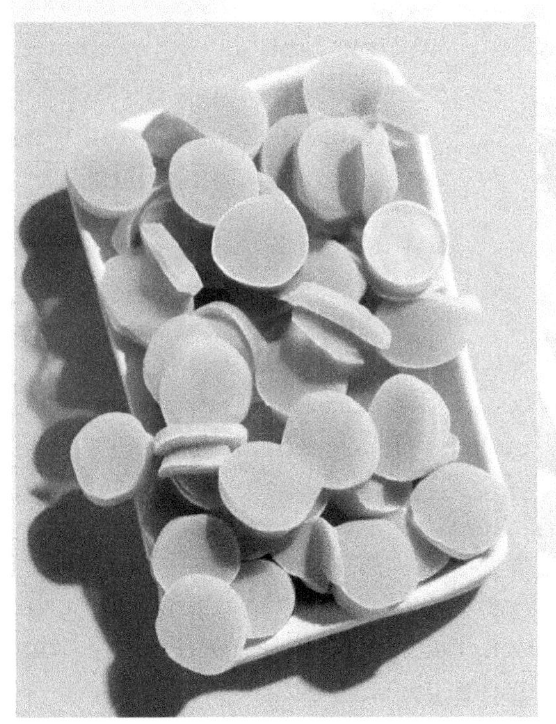

Time of Preparation: 45 minutes

Serving Unit: 1 lozenge

Ingredients:

- 1/2 cup water
- 1 tablespoon dried licorice root
- 1/2 cup honey
- 1/2 cup powdered sugar (for dusting)

Procedures:

1. Prepare Licorice Infusion: In a small saucepan, bring 1/2 cup of water to a boil. Add dried

licorice root to the boiling water, reduce heat, and let it simmer for 20-30 minutes until the liquid is reduced by half.

2. Strain and Cool: Remove the saucepan from heat and strain the licorice infusion using a fine mesh sieve or cheesecloth to remove the licorice root pieces. Allow the liquid to cool slightly.

3. Add Honey: While the licorice infusion is still warm (not boiling), stir in 1/2 cup of honey until fully dissolved.

4. Forming Lozenges: Pour the honey and licorice mixture onto a clean, flat surface dusted with powdered sugar. Use a spatula to spread the mixture evenly to about 1/4 inch thickness.

5. Cutting Lozenges: Use a sharp knife or pizza cutter to cut the mixture into small lozenge-sized pieces. Dust each piece with powdered sugar to prevent sticking.

6. Cool and Store: Allow the lozenges to cool completely at room temperature until firm. Store in an airtight container layered with parchment paper or wax paper to prevent sticking.

Tips and Tricks:

➢ Use organic licorice root to avoid pesticides and chemicals.

➢ Adjust the thickness of the mixture to create lozenges of desired size and thickness.

➢ Store the lozenges in a cool, dry place away from direct sunlight to maintain freshness and effectiveness.

Nutritional Value (per serving - 1 lozenge):

➢ Calories: 10
➢ Carbohydrates: 3g
➢ Sugar: 3g

Health Benefits:

➢ Sore Throat Relief: Licorice root has demulcent properties that help soothe and coat the throat, providing relief from soreness and irritation.

➢ Anti-inflammatory: Contains glycyrrhizin and flavonoids that exhibit anti-inflammatory effects, reducing swelling and discomfort.

➢ Antioxidant: Provides antioxidant support to the immune system, promoting overall health and well-being.

Storage and Heating Requirements:

Storage: Keep the licorice root throat lozenges in an airtight container in a cool, dry place. Use within 2-3 months for optimal freshness and effectiveness.

Heating: Serve at room temperature. Avoid heating to preserve the beneficial properties of licorice root and honey.

Enjoy your Licorice Root Throat Lozenges as a soothing and effective remedy for sore throats and respiratory comfort. Incorporate them into your daily routine or use as needed for natural throat relief and immune support.

Recipes for Immune Support:

Welcome to Recipes for Immune Support, where we explore the nourishing power of ingredients crafted into wholesome remedies for your well-being. In this collection, we delve into the world of natural immunity boosters, from soothing teas that fortify defenses to nutrient-rich soups that rejuvenate the body. Each recipe is designed to support your immune system with the goodness of whole foods and herbal remedies, providing a holistic approach to health and vitality. Join me on this journey to discover simple yet effective ways to strengthen your immune system naturally, ensuring you thrive year-round with the benefits of homemade immune-supporting recipes.

Elderberry Syrup

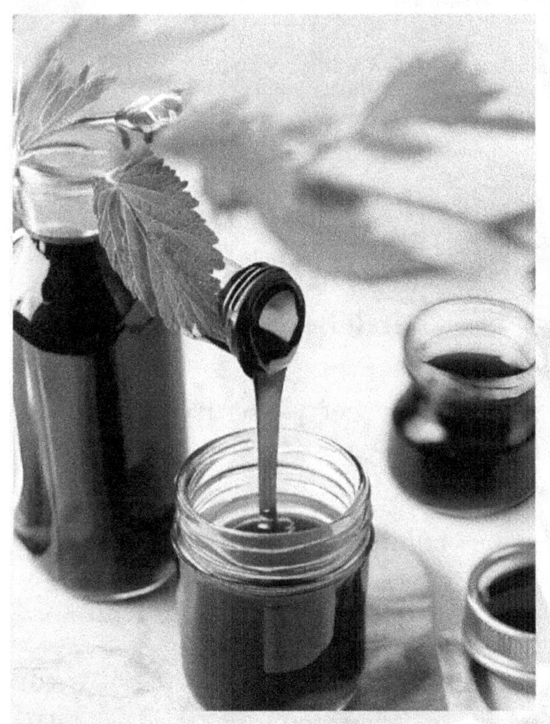

Time of Preparation: **45** minutes

Serving Unit: 1 tablespoon

Ingredients:

- ➢ 1 cup dried elderberries (or 2 cups fresh elderberries)
- ➢ 3 cups water
- ➢ 1 cup honey (or maple syrup for a vegan option)
- ➢ Optional: 1-2 cinnamon sticks, 1 inch of fresh ginger (sliced), 4-6 whole cloves

Procedures:

Prepare Elderberry Infusion:

1. In a medium saucepan, combine the dried elderberries (or fresh elderberries) and water.
2. Add optional spices like cinnamon sticks, fresh ginger, and whole cloves for

additional flavor and health benefits.

3. Bring the mixture to a boil, then reduce heat and let it simmer uncovered for 30-45 minutes until the liquid is reduced by half.

Strain and Cool:

4. Remove the saucepan from heat and let the mixture cool slightly.
5. Strain the elderberry mixture through a fine mesh sieve or cheesecloth into a clean bowl, pressing gently to extract all liquid.

Add Sweetener:

6. While the elderberry liquid is still warm (not boiling), stir in honey or maple syrup until fully dissolved.
7. Adjust sweetness to taste preference, keeping in mind that honey adds additional health benefits.

Cool and Store:

8. Allow the elderberry syrup to cool completely at room temperature.
9. Pour the syrup into clean, sterilized glass bottles or jars with airtight lids for storage.

Tips and Tricks:

➢ Use dried elderberries for convenience or fresh elderberries when in season for a more vibrant flavor.
➢ Incorporate optional spices like cinnamon, ginger, and cloves to enhance taste and provide additional immune-boosting properties.
➢ Store elderberry syrup in the refrigerator to maintain freshness. Use within 2-3 months for optimal potency.

Nutritional Value (per serving - 1 tablespoon):

➢ Calories: **45**
➢ Carbohydrates: **12g**
➢ Sugar: **10g**

Health Benefits:

➢ Immune Support: Elderberries are rich in antioxidants and vitamins that help boost the immune system and fight off colds and flu.
➢ Anti-inflammatory: Contains compounds that reduce inflammation and promote overall health.
➢ Respiratory Health: Elderberry syrup may help alleviate symptoms of respiratory infections and allergies.

Storage and Heating Requirements:

➢ Storage: Keep elderberry syrup refrigerated in sealed glass containers to preserve freshness and potency.

➢ **Heating:** Serve elderberry syrup at room temperature or slightly warmed. Avoid boiling or excessive heat to maintain its beneficial properties.

Enjoy your Elderberry Syrup as a delicious and nutritious addition to your wellness routine, supporting immune health with the natural goodness of elderberries and optional spices. Incorporate it daily during cold and flu season or as needed to boost your body's defenses naturally.

Garlic Honey Elixir

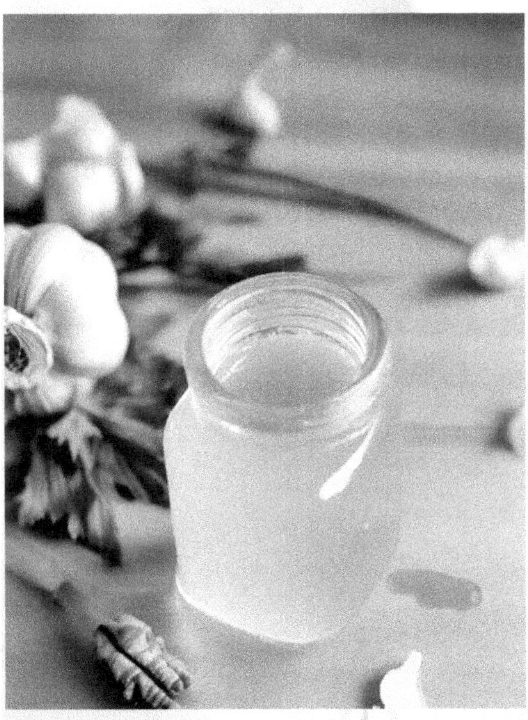

Time of Preparation: 10 minutes

Serving Unit: 1 teaspoon

Ingredients:

➢ 1/2 cup raw honey
➢ 8-10 cloves garlic, peeled and crushed

Procedures:

Prepare Garlic Infusion:

1. In a clean, sterilized glass jar, combine the raw honey with crushed garlic cloves.
2. Stir well to ensure all garlic cloves are coated with honey.

Infuse and Store:

3. Seal the jar tightly and store it in a cool, dark place for 3-5 days to allow the garlic to infuse into the honey.

Strain (optional):

4. After 3-5 days, strain the garlic pieces from the honey using a fine mesh sieve or cheesecloth if desired, although leaving the garlic pieces in can enhance the potency.

Tips and Tricks:

➢ Use raw, organic honey for its antimicrobial and soothing properties.
➢ Crush garlic cloves slightly to release their beneficial compounds before adding to honey.

> Adjust the amount of garlic based on personal preference and tolerance.

Nutritional Value (per serving - 1 teaspoon):

> Calories: 20
> Carbohydrates: 5g
> Sugar: 5g

Health Benefits:

> Immune Support: Garlic is rich in allicin and other compounds known to support the immune system and ward off infections.
> Antioxidant: Honey provides antioxidants that help combat free radicals and promote overall health.
> Respiratory Health: Garlic honey elixir may help alleviate symptoms of colds, coughs, and sore throats.

Storage and Heating Requirements:

> Storage: Keep the garlic honey elixir in a sealed glass jar at room temperature. Use within 1-2 months for optimal flavor and effectiveness.
> Heating: Serve the elixir at room temperature. Avoid heating to preserve the beneficial properties of both garlic and honey.

Enjoy your Garlic Honey Elixir as a natural remedy to support immune health and alleviate respiratory discomfort. Incorporate it into your daily routine during cold and flu season or as needed for its soothing and immune-boosting benefits, harnessing the power of garlic and honey in this simple yet potent elixir.

Turmeric Golden Milk

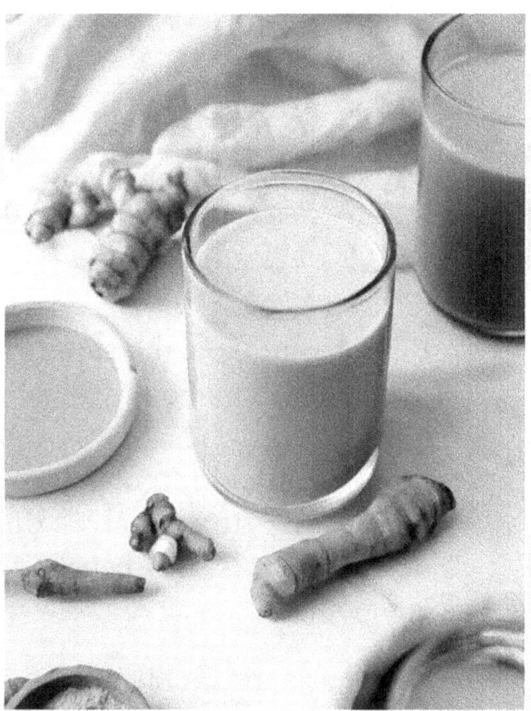

Time of Preparation: 10 minutes

Serving Unit: 1 cup

Ingredients:

- 2 cups milk (dairy or plant-based like almond, coconut, or oat milk)
- 1 teaspoon ground turmeric
- 1/2 teaspoon ground cinnamon
- 1/4 teaspoon ground ginger (or 1/2 inch fresh ginger, grated)
- 1 pinch ground black pepper
- 1 tablespoon honey or maple syrup (optional, for sweetness)
- 1 tablespoon coconut oil or ghee (optional, for creaminess)

Procedures:

Mixing the Ingredients:

1. In a small saucepan, heat the milk over medium-low heat until it is warm but not boiling.
2. Add ground turmeric, cinnamon, ginger, and a pinch of black pepper to the milk.
3. Stir continuously to combine the ingredients and prevent any lumps from forming.

Simmering and Straining (optional):

4. Simmer the mixture gently for about 5 minutes to allow the flavors to meld together.
5. If using fresh ginger, simmer for an additional 2-3 minutes.
6. Optionally, strain the golden milk through a fine mesh sieve to remove any solid particles.

Sweetening (optional):

7. Add honey or maple syrup to sweeten the golden milk, if desired. Stir until fully dissolved.

Adding Fat (optional):

8. For added creaminess, stir in coconut oil or ghee until melted and well incorporated.

Serve:

9. Pour the turmeric golden milk into mugs and serve warm.

Tips and Tricks:

- Use freshly ground spices for the best flavor and health benefits.
- Adjust the sweetness to your taste preference with honey or maple syrup.
- Including a pinch of black pepper enhances the absorption of turmeric's active compound, curcumin.

Nutritional Value (per serving - 1 cup):

- Calories: 150
- Carbohydrates: 15g
- Sugar: 12g
- Protein: 5g
- Fat: 7g

Health Benefits:

- Anti-inflammatory: Turmeric and ginger contain compounds that help reduce inflammation in the body.
- Antioxidant: Cinnamon and turmeric are rich in antioxidants that combat oxidative stress.
- Digestive Health: Ginger aids digestion and can alleviate nausea.

Storage and Heating Requirements:

- Storage: Store any leftover turmeric golden milk in a sealed container in the refrigerator for up to 2 days. Reheat gently on the stovetop or in the microwave until warmed through.
- Heating: Avoid boiling or overheating to preserve the delicate flavors and beneficial compounds.

Enjoy your Turmeric Golden Milk as a comforting and nutritious beverage, perfect for promoting overall health and well-being with its blend of warming spices and healthful ingredients. Incorporate it into your daily routine to reap the numerous benefits of turmeric and spices in a soothing and delicious form.

Conclusion

In conclusion, this book on herbalism serves as a comprehensive guide for beginners and enthusiasts alike, embarking on a journey through the rich and diverse world of herbal medicine and culinary arts. Throughout its pages, we have explored the foundational principles of herbalism, from understanding the historical roots and philosophical underpinnings to navigating the benefits and potential risks of herbal remedies.

We have delved into the dual perspectives of traditional herbal knowledge and modern scientific approaches, bridging ancient wisdom with contemporary understanding to offer a holistic view of herbal medicine today. Each chapter has unfolded with practical insights and detailed guidance, empowering readers to cultivate their understanding of herbs, their cultivation, identification, and sustainable harvesting practices.

The exploration of various medicinal plants—from Aloe Vera to Turmeric, from culinary herbs like Basil and Oregano to medicinal powerhouses such as Echinacea and Valerian—has provided a deep dive into their unique properties, cultivation methods, and diverse therapeutic uses.

Practical sections on preparation methods, safety considerations, and herbal recipes for common ailments have equipped readers with the tools needed to incorporate herbal remedies into everyday life responsibly and effectively. Whether crafting herbal teas and infusions for relaxation, preparing soothing salves and syrups for health support, or simply enhancing culinary creations with herbal infusions and sauces, this book has aimed to inspire and empower.

In closing, the journey through this book is not just a study of plants but an invitation to connect with nature's healing gifts and harness their potential for wellness and vitality. By embracing the knowledge shared within these pages, readers are encouraged to explore, experiment, and integrate herbs into their lifestyles mindfully, fostering a deeper connection to the natural world and reaping the benefits of herbal medicine for years to come.

May this book serve as a companion and guide, fostering a lifelong passion for herbalism and inspiring a journey of discovery, health, and harmony with nature.